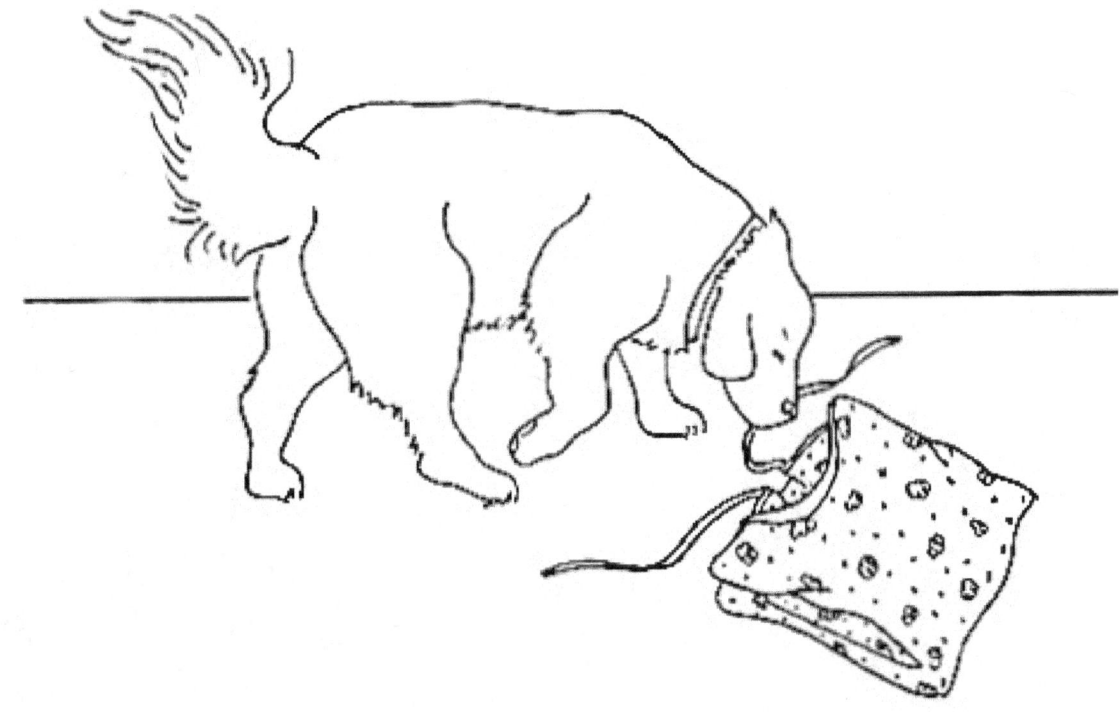

What to Expect When...

SAYING GOOD-BYE TO YOUR PROSTATE

How to Beat Prostate Cancer,
Ease Your Mind,
and Laugh While Doing It

by

Jamie MacKenzie

with

Illustrations

by

Lisa Schwartz

For Ed, Cheryl, David, Cordis & Thayer

...and for Caleb, Zuzu & Anio

And in loving memory
of Laura, Sasha, Cris...

...and Trip

CONTENTS

ACKNOWLEDGMENTS

I must first admit that I hate reading acknowledgments in books. I get impatient and want to dive in without the fuss of reading about "everyone who made this possible, blah, blah, blah..." Then if I don't read them I often feel a sense of guilt. Go figure. I'm a Pisces.

But now it's my book I've just finished writing, and all I see are the many faces of loved ones and colleagues who kept the faith while I was terrified and lonely, who prayed and chanted for me, who kept me in their thoughts daily, who reached out and checked in on me, who cried with me and who made me laugh, who took care of my four-legged children and offered wonderful suggestions - and who, above all, encouraged me to take the leap of faith far into the unknown and uncertain, assuring me all the while that they would ALWAYS be there to catch me.

All of you know who you are - especially the Tower Hill School Class of 1970 - along with the many wonderful doctors and their kind staffs.

Knowing that I wanted this book to be 'user-friendly' and disarming, Andy Pyle shrewdly introduced me to Lisa Schwartz and her terrific illustrations - and to Kurt Swanson who kept us all calm and on keel.

Elliott Robinson. Designer and UltraGeek, who solves all technical design problems instantly. An amazing, endlessly generous friend. Always there to lend a hand.

Josie Jesser, who handed me to Quintin Springstead who conquered very stubborn and complex formatting issues, and is the soul of patience.

Brenda Barrier. Neighbor, friend, diligent editor, and mother to the endlessly entertaining Flying Nicholas, her German Shorthaired Pointer - I adore you.

Adam Slevin. My surgeon's physician assistant, and a kind friend who somehow found time in his hectic life to help advise.

Paddy and Jim Rossbach. No one could have finer next-door neighbors and supportive friends.

Wendy Goidell and Phantom. Tremendous thanks for 'stabilizing' me when I needed it most.

Dr. Ward 'Trip' Casscells. Literally, my first friend. We were born on the same day, in the same hospital, nearly at the same hour. Both with red hair. No one could have a finer 'twin'. A remarkable soul and brave advocate.

And without my pal Thom Mozloom, saying, "Hey brother, you gotta riff on this stuff," there wouldn't be a book at all. Thanks, Bro.

And lastly, Ed Deci - an extraordinary human being, patient teacher, brilliant theorist and writer - my Rock of Gibralter.

My deepest thanks to all of you friends, and heartfelt, best wishes to all the strangers reading this - the men facing this journey, and the men and women in their lives supporting them.

Jamie MacKenzie - Taconic, Connecticut

P.S. The book has been formatted in large print. The last thing you want to be told, when diagnosed, is that you also need reading glasses!

This book is not intended as a substitute for the medical advice of physicians. The reader should regularly consult a physician in all matters relating to his or her health, and particularly in respect to any symptoms that may require diagnosis or medical attention.

PREFACE

This book is not just for men everywhere over 35. It is also for younger men who are or will be the sons or brothers, nephews, partners or friends to someone with prostate cancer. It is for women of all ages who are or will be the wives or daughters, sisters, nieces or friends of someone with prostate cancer.

Prostate cancer screenings (PSA tests) are not just for men over 50 anymore. Three out of ten men will develop prostate disease by age 70. It is the most common, most treatable and curable cancer we will have.

Any cancer diagnosis is a terrifying one. This handbook memoir, written by a prostate cancer survivor, walks men and their loved ones through every step before them - from PSA numbers climbing to biopsy, from diagnosis to pre-op, from surgery to recovery - all while telling the reader not only what to expect, but also showing them how to mine and benefit from the inherent humor that will unexpectedly and mercifully accompany the fear.

MONITORING YOUR PSA NUMBERS FAITHFULLY

The first thing that must be said is that although the PSA test can be an imperfect one, it saves lives. Period. You don't have to have a complete physical. A four minute blood draw and a digital rectal examination. Total: four minutes and ten seconds! You don't have to spend a lot of money. The PSA results will give you and your doctor a baseline which, as you grow older, may or may not rise. But you must have a baseline to begin to protect yourself.

Many now feel that PSA testing should begin at age 35. There was a 38 year-old in my group of fellow patients. Need I say more?

If you're reading this book, either you or your loved one most likely has a baseline in place; perhaps one that has risen, perhaps one that has not. In either case, you or he has a baseline - and this is good.

A terrific tool to use has been designed and is located online at: WWW.PROSTATETRACKER.ORG

This lets you set up a completely discreet account and charts your PSA results from testing to testing. It even has a reminder that emails you when it is time to have your next test. It is private. It is free. And it is empowering.

What to Expect When...

SAYING GOOD-BYE TO YOUR PROSTATE

How to Beat Prostate Cancer,
Ease Your Mind,
and Laugh While Doing It

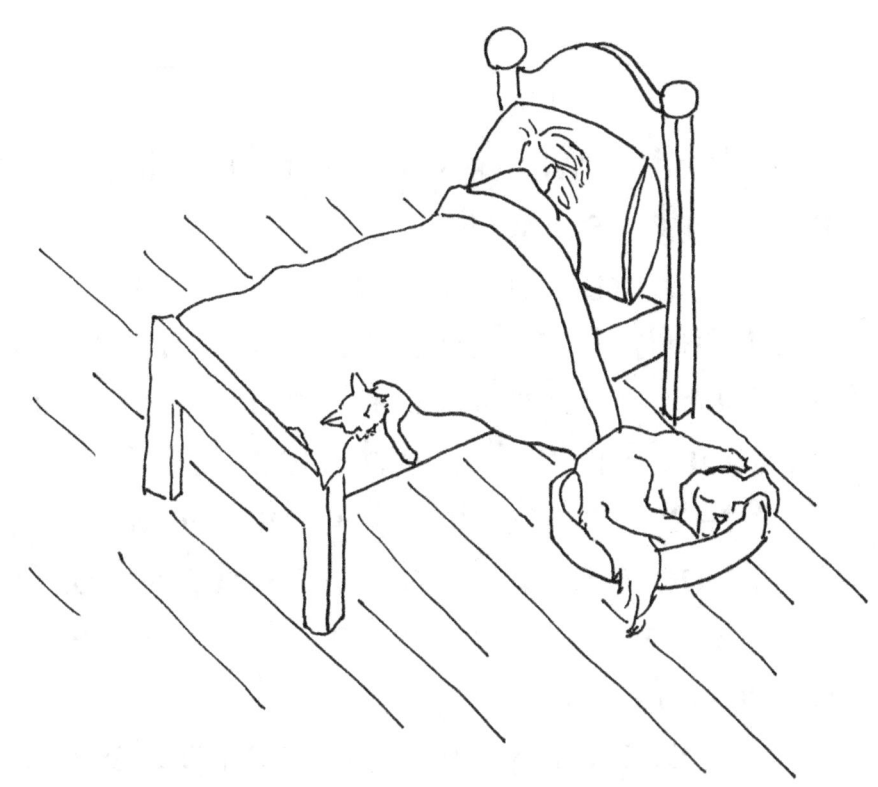

Chapter 1

THE DREAM

Early January. Last year. I awoke from a dream where I had been visiting the home of a childhood friend. We were present-day grownups, and she had inherited her parents' house.

As I walked through the house, around every corner, I was greeted by a childhood schoolmate who welcomed me with open arms and lovingly called my name. There were David, Lane, Debbie, Genelle, Craig, Nicky, Donny, Libby, Mina, Sydney, Carol, Ginny, Wendy, Trip, Rory, J.O., Lisa, Rachel, Larry, Judy, Frank, Bruce, and on and on. The warmth was almost overwhelming. And simply blissful. I was glowing with affirmation and love, and resisted waking up as long as I could.

Showered, fed the cats and the pooch, and sat down to meditate before breakfast, as I have done for more than thirty years. During the meditation, I heard my email alert bell sound once. I would check it after I finished meditating.

Bread in the toaster, and I walked into my office to check the overnight emails. At the top of the list read the subject line, *Craig E. Looking for Jamie MacKenzie from Tower Hill School.*

I rubbed my eyes in complete disbelief, opened the email and read that two childhood classmates were trying to find me, and asked if I would reply. Now this sort of thing has happened before in my dreams and meditations, but never so precisely flowing from a dreamscape to reality.

I emailed back immediately, and within thirty-six hours I was having hour-long conversations with classmates I hadn't seen or spoken to for more than forty years. Each conversation, without exception, was effortless and breezy, as if it had only been the length of a study-hall period since we last conversed.

Things snowballed from that point as more classmates emailed and called. It was remarkable - the flood of warmth and affection and love. I realized, as my bliss continued, that these 'children' were really the first family I'd had outside my own family. We started at four years old, together in pre-kindergarten. There were twelve of us. Running, crayoning, squabbling, jumping, snacking, peeing, singing - and after it all, napping on the floor, safely curled up on our blankets for Rest Time.

Bonds that would run through a lifetime were formed there, quietly, with unseen, tremendous certainty while we sucked our thumbs and snuggled close to each other.

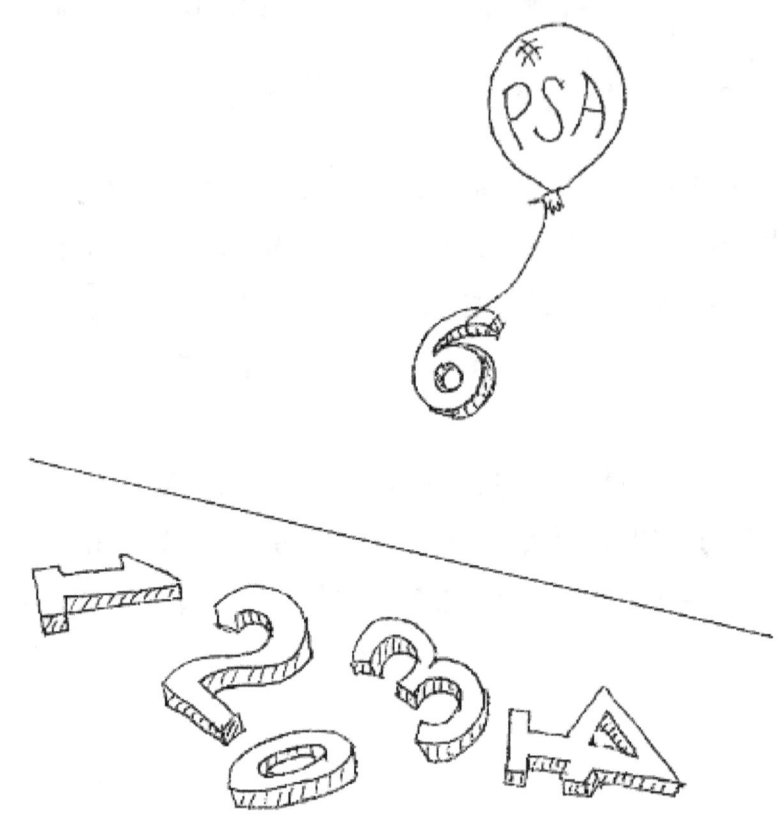

Chapter 2

WHAT TO DO
IF PSA
NUMBERS RISE

Less than a month after the blissful dream which harkened the reuniting of the four-year olds, now fifty-eight, my doctor, following my physical, commented that my PSA numbers had risen over the past two years.

"What does PSA stand for, Kristie?" I asked her.

Prostate Specific Antigens. Okay. Now what to do? She recommended I see a local urologist who would prescribe ten days of an antibiotic which would likely drop my numbers indicating that I had chronic prostatitis.

The local urologist did a digital examination. He found my prostate gland to be slightly enlarged and did put me on the medication for ten days. Medication which, by the way, cost thirteen dollars a pill AFTER insurance. And I have very good prescription insurance. A hundred and thirty dollars later, my wallet was empty, but my PSA count had only gone down a quarter of a point, from 6 to 5.75. I was disappointed to be certain, but not at all alarmed - especially when he recommended taking two months of ciprofloxacin and then testing again.

After reading up about Cipro, on the internet, and finding that it can cause deterioration of the Achilles tendon, my stomach began to turn. Something wasn't as it should be. I knew I didn't want to do two months of a potentially damaging drug. And that wonderful old signal went off in my gut: time to go to the big city. New York City. I had lived there for twenty-six years and was accustomed to getting the best medical help one could. I was not going to leave this to an affable but, as it turned out, decidedly inept urologist.

Many phone calls ensued to friends in the city who recommended a number of urologists. I settled on one, and took the train in to see him the next week. He examined me and took another PSA test. He also asked the most important question: had my urologist, in the country, broken the PSA total down into 'free' versus 'bound'? I phoned them from his office and found they had not. Even his secretary was unsure what the terms meant at first. The New York doctor told me that breaking the PSA numbers down into 'free' versus 'bound' is really the best way to get information out of a good, but not perfect, testing system.

He continued. If the free and bound numbers are in parity, things are likely all right, and a 'watchful wait' is recommended. In that case, you continue testing every month in the watchful mode. If the numbers, on the other hand, are out of proportion, then they strongly recommend getting a biopsy.

A week later he phoned to say my numbers were 17% to 83%. This was the first of many out-of-body moments I experienced. I found myself drifting upward, and hovering slightly above myself trying to catch my breath. This can't be happening to me, I of course thought. Yes, my father had had a slight case of colon cancer, successfully treated. I'd had a clean bill of health colonoscopy two years earlier, and I knew of no incidence of prostate cancer in my family.

I was brought back down to Earth when he turned me over to his bookkeeper who informed me that he didn't participate with insurance plans, and that the fee for the biopsy would be $3,400. Half down before, and the balance due after the biopsy.

This was going to be very difficult for me to swing.

At neighbors, a couple of nights later for dinner and support, I mentioned how expensive the Manhattan biopsy would be and that none of it would be covered by insurance. Paddy, the wife, leapt to her feet, saying she'd be right back. After a few moments, she returned with a printout of pages from her computer.

"Here's the guy you should look up in the city. I used to work there. Give him a call." I beamed thanks at her. Girl Power had started kicking in.

It turned out that her recommendation was not a urologist who did biopsies, but an oncologist treating cancer patients. His assistant recommended one of the heads of the urology department at his hospital, and I telephoned his office. After being told he was covered by insurance, I sighed with some relief. It seemed, after speaking with his bookkeeper, that I would only be out about $500 for the procedure.

So back into the city I went. The head urologist's intern did a digital rectal exam, then asked me to fill out pages - and I mean pages - of questions about my penis and erections and sex life. Be prepared to laugh. I didn't know there could be more than a couple of questions about one's erection. I swear they write these penile questionnaires to purposely cause mirth, and it worked - at least for me. It was the first time I laughed since all this began. And I was grateful. After this, the doctor came in and explained to me what a biopsy would entail.

Now here's where a parallel universe sets in. In your diagnostic journey with Mr. Prostate, every other word used in conversation or explanation will be taken as a pun and usually a bad one. Entail. See? I already did it and I'm only on page eight. Don't worry, there will be many more, I assure you. And the thing is, don't try to avoid it. God, in her great wisdom - and I do think of God as being the beloved actress, Hattie McDaniel, from *Gone With the Wind* - has arranged this to KEEP YOU LAUGHING. It will save you. It will lift and distract you. And it will promote blood circulation down there where you need it for healing.

After looking at my results, the urologist and his intern agreed that a biopsy should be done. It was scheduled for March 18th. This was a really insulting birthday present to be looking forward to. Especially as every time I spoke or visited their offices, they started each conversation with, "What is your birth date, please, Mr. MacKenzie?" When they arranged for the biopsy to be done on my actual birthday, I figured it was in case one or the other of us had forgotten my birth date. Scheduling the procedure on that day would make it ever so much easier for all involved.

Three weeks went by, and the day loomed. I asked a friend, who was going to be in the city anyway, to collect me after the biopsy to accompany me home on the two-hour train ride to the country. She caringly obliged and was able to be there as I was checked in and later released.

As fate would have it, I was caught behind a school bus on the way to the train station. With literally three minutes to spare, I passed a car in front of me on the last straight-away before the station, and turned against the red arrow traffic light. Pulling into a parking place, I opened my door and was greeted by a town policeman whose vehicle had me pinned in like a scene from *Kojak* - without the bad music.

"Do you have any idea how fast you were going!? You must have been going more than eighty!" he barked at me. "And you went through the red indicator!! License and registration!"

As my hands fumbled in the glove compartment for the elusive registration, I told him I knew what I'd done - that I was trying to make the train because I was going into the city for a prostate biopsy. I looked up and the train was mercifully still at the platform. Then I started to fall apart. I began to shake, and my chin trembled noticeably. I finally found my registration. After some quick paperwork in his car, he returned with a ticket hastily filled out and said, "Go make your train," then, taking my hand in both of his, he added, "and good luck!"

I ran, made the train as the doors were closing, found a seat way at the far end of an empty car, and began sobbing.

After a couple of stops, I heard the familiar voice of my favorite conductor, Tim. I raised my hand, and hollered "Guilty as charged."

"That was you with the cop!?"

"Yep," and I explained how I earned the ticket.

"Oh, shit - we all go through that light when we're running late! Shit!"

Then I blurted, "Tim, I didn't have time to buy a ticket."

"Oh well, I'll sell you one - and to me, you're looking like a senior citizen, so just give me ten bucks, amigo." Although I was only eight hours in to turning fifty-nine, I certainly felt like a senior citizen at that moment.

When I realized that I had not, of course, had the time to pay for the day's parking, Tim asked me what space number my car was in, and told me that on the way back up, in an hour, he would purchase the receipt and tuck it under my windshield wiper.

Tim's unique blend of wicked humor, Bolshevik leftism, and totally unexpected generosity calmed me down. I told him what was happening that day. As we parted, he wished me luck, blew me a kiss followed by a huge smile, and said he hoped I'd make the earlier afternoon return train that he would be working on.

The policeman. Tim. My neighbors. Childhood classmates. Angels were gathering, armed with powerful weapons of caring and support.

IMPORTANT NOTE: Again, PSA testing is not perfect. Nothing is. A digital examination is also crucial in helping to determine what may or may not be going on in the prostate. A friend's disease was detected by his doctor's mercifully sensitive fingertip - not just an enlargement of the gland, but slight anomalies present to the touch - even though his PSA was low and had not moved a jot. That said, the PSA test helped save my life, and both tests should begin at age 35.

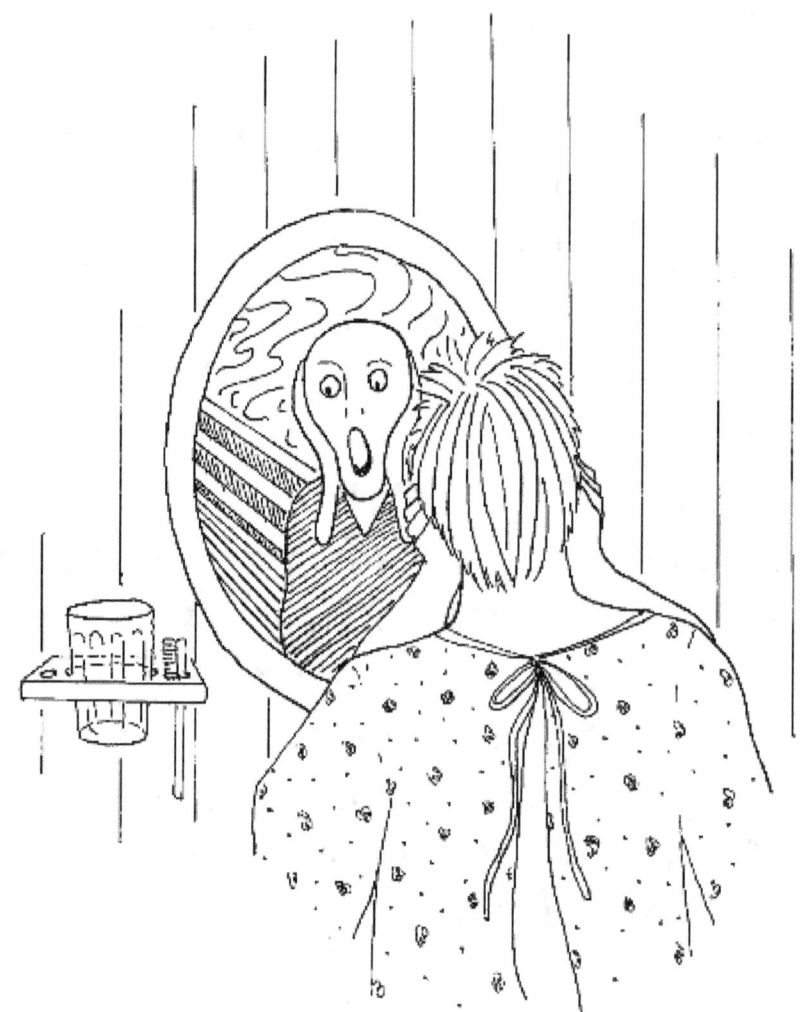

Chapter 3

**FACING
A BIOPSY**

Even the most delicately explained, empathetically spoken, description of a prostate biopsy will instantly cause the mind to concoct the darkest of fantasies. The reality, however, is quite different. I'm not saying it will be a cakewalk, but it is so much easier and less painful than one imagines it to be.

Okay. So you'll be told by your doctor that a 'wand' will be inserted into your rectum, and that an ultrasound will be read by a technician before the actual biopsy is performed. The room I was in was dark and warm. With only the hospital gown covering my front and shoulders, I lay on my left side. The ultrasound technician applied some lubricant to my backside and the wand was gradually inserted.

Now the sheer thought of this, when explained by the doctor, is where many men simply freak out. Okay, freak out for a moment or two. I'll even give you three moments. Then stop and grow up. This is your body. This is technology helping your body, potentially saving your life. Put it into perspective. These people are dedicated to helping you. So be a good team member (there it is again, I told you) and breathe.

It is small. It has been warmed.

And it will not - I repeat - will not turn you gay.

After about five minutes of ultrasound, the technician told me the doctor would be right in. I thanked him and asked him how things looked on his monitor. He replied, "They look good."

I smiled and thought, okay, this is all going to be all right. It's good I'm having the biopsy, but things are going to be all right.

My doctor entered the room, greeted me, sat down beside me and explained that inside the wand that was still in my rectum, was a chamber where a needle would be guided. This is the instrument that takes sample plugs of the prostate gland for testing.

As my friend Joe stated, "You know, the argument against Intelligent Design is, in fact, the prostate." And he's right. It does its job well, but it is located in a very difficult place to reach. The good news is that, yes, they have a solution. But brace yourself, laddie - the bad news is that it is through the rectal wall.

That's right. The rectal wall. Tell me when I should continue. I'll give you a little time.

Okay?

You're doing great.

So the wand within the wand has a triggering device which shoots a hollow needle through the rectal wall and into pre-designated areas of the prostate gland determined by the ultrasound results. It is then retracted, and each plug taken is stored for testing.

Then the biopsy doctor, who I must add, is an elegant older gentleman with an exquisitely soft and comforting voice, calmly whispered, "Now you're going to feel two little pricks..."

It was only in retrospect that I recalled this and started laughing myself silly. I have retold that moment scores of times since my surgery and it never fails to crack me or the listener up.

And these are the moments you will cherish as you recover from the daunting complexity of emotions on The Journey.

The noise made by the triggering device is, in fact, far more disconcerting than anything you feel. It was jarringly loud. I almost jumped, which is hard to do when lying on one's side. Instead of the "two little pricks" warning, I would substitute, "You're going to hear a sharp bang." (Sorry - not as funny as the other puns, granted, but there it is.) The subsequent bangs were fine because I was accustomed to the sound. In a few minutes, it was all over and I was walking out of the office wearing my first pair of disposable pull-ups. I had been advised to bring them along for the train ride home.

My companion and I navigated through the NYC subway up to the 125th Street station to make our commuter train back to Connecticut. It was sufficiently crowded that we had to stand for the first half hour. This was not a problem as I felt a little tender down under. We got talking with a fellow passenger, a documentary filmmaker, and the next thing I knew I told him of the day's event. He was very sympathetic, and kind and has since become a friend. I found I was already determined to be a poster boy for spreading the word. I'm not sure why, but I wanted to tell every man and woman on the train.

By the time we changed over to the extension train for the second hour's ride home, I'd found a place to sit and tried to snooze. Unable to, I unfolded a discarded *New York Times* on the seat next to me. After some cursory glances, my eyes fell upon the title, "Dildos Come Out of the Closet."

It was a full page article about the history of dildos, relieving anxiety in nervous Victorian women, and how they are sold everywhere these days - with no plain brown wrapper needed. And there was a photograph of a husband and wife, sitting in a physician's office, with the caption "Jim G. and his wife of Tenafly, New Jersey, have a mold made of his erection before having prostate surgery, to create a dildo for his wife."

I certainly was in no doubt that the universe was acknowledging my path, more and more, in unexpected ways.

As I continued chuckling about this, Tim, the conductor, came shuffling down the aisle of the last car saying, "I'm looking for Jamie. I'm looking for Jamie. Where IS he!?" I raised my hand, and he came up and asked how everything had gone. I said okay, and he handed me a brown bag. "This is for you. I'm going to collect the tickets. I'll be back.

Don't open it." Off he went. I resisted opening the bag until he returned about five minutes later.

Sitting down, Tim said, "Go ahead - now you can open it."

In the bag were two cups of coffee, one for each of us, but there was something else larger. I pulled out a plastic container. Through the clear-domed top I saw a slice of cake with one rainbow colored candle on it.

"Happy Birthday!" Tim loudly saluted. I beamed from ear to ear. The thought that he would take the time on his lunch break to pay my parking fee, put the receipt under the windshield wiper, and pick up a slice of cake making sure there was a candle on it, simply dissolved me into a state of pure joy. I could just hear him yelling out across the deli's counter, during his lunch break, "Hey, Myrtle! Give me a piece of cake for my pal, Jamie - and put a candle on it!"

Hands down, the best birthday of my life.

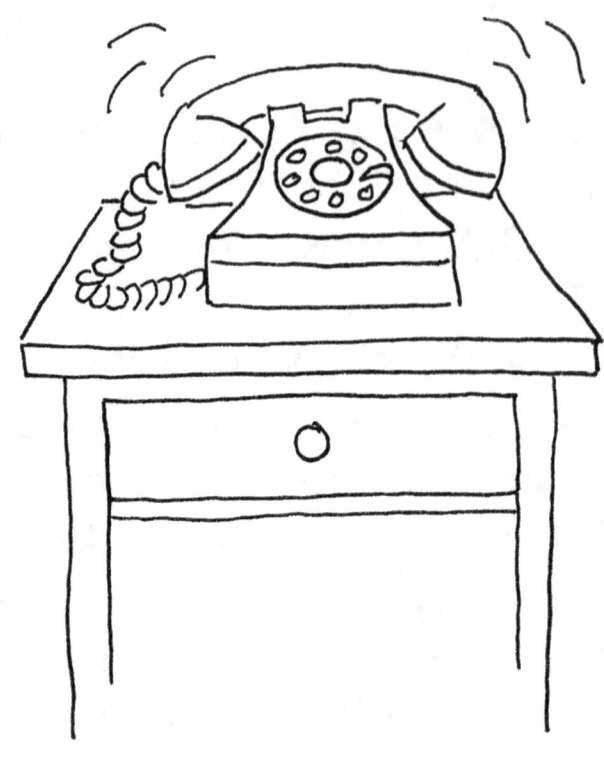

Chapter 4

THE AGONIZING WAIT
FOR RESULTS

Okay, so now you have to wait for the biopsy results. This is going to be the hardest thing you'll go through. All you can see lying before you is the Unknown. The unforgiving, uncompassionate, and silent Unknown. For almost ten days, in my case, because my procedure was done on a Friday. So I would not have results until the second Monday.

Difficult to foretell, I suspect, because each of us is different, but suffice it to say you will think of nothing else but what the results might be. Some hours and days will be better than others, but most of it will be hell. Thank God I've been meditating for nearly thirty-five years. For an hour or so a day, at least, I was able to keep my head from blowing off my shoulders in anxiety.

Although I never really grasped the concept of the results showing disease - I was fine, everything's going to be great - I nonetheless couldn't really function very well. And that's simply what you have to accept. That this stage will be the most difficult. The most lonely stage. And that you will get through it.

Not surprisingly, my four-legged 'kids' - two cats, Caleb and Zuzu, and my Golden Retriever, Anio - came to the rescue. The more anxiety I felt and demonstrated, the more attentive and loving they became. So much so that both cats made a point of sleeping on my bed, which they heretofore had only done irregularly, alongside me and Anio. Every morning they each licked my nose as long as I could tolerate their sandpaper tongues. They kissed my ears. They kissed my eyebrows. They kissed my nose and my chin. They each routinely buttressed my backside, uncomplainingly accommodating my turning from side to side during the night. And through it all, Caleb made sure that when I was lying on my side, facing him, he was right there letting me hold his paw in my fingers. This got me through many a near sleepless night. I'd awaken hours later and still be holding his paw. An old friend calls them furry angels. And that they are.

Many will choose to read everything they can get their hands on: online, in books and magazines. I tried this for a while but it only served to make me more anxious. You just have to wait. And besides which, I was cautioned by my local doctor, Kristie, to take everything I read online with a block of salt.

The biopsy doctor's office sent me home with a pamphlet about what to expect after the procedure. A little tenderness here, a little blood in the urine. Perhaps some in your stool. And that my semen might appear a little 'rusty'. That was about it.

The first time I 'self-stimulated' after the biopsy - and yes, that's what they call it - I was relieved and horrified. My orgasm was normal but the ejaculate did not appear rusty, it was a very dark red - almost black. In a bit of a panic, I rang the doctor's office. The nurse allayed my fears, casually adding, "You know, they really should redo that pamphlet."

Thank you...

So don't worry if your semen is brilliantly dark red or rusty. This is simply because the plugs taken through the wall of the rectum cause bleeding and this collects in the seminal fluid. It is natural. It is a total surprise. And a very discomforting one after a lifetime of seeing a different color.

The more sex or self-stimulation you have, the more it will return to its natural color.

Don't worry. Just enjoy yourself.

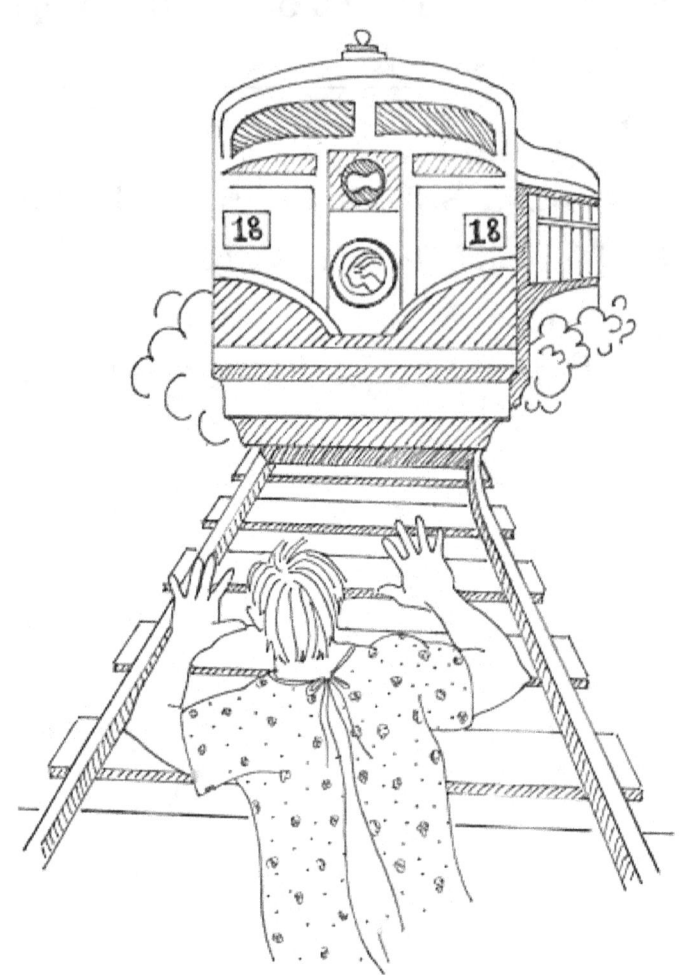

Chapter 5

<u>ACCEPTING</u>
<u>THE DIAGNOSIS</u>

When the second Monday came, I rang my local doctor, Kristie. She'd had no word from NYC. I was hoping that this meant that I was in the clear. Of course I would be. After all, I hadn't been in the hospital since I was five years old for a tonsillectomy. It was all going to be fine. I felt confident enough to telephone the biopsy doctor's office for the results instead of waiting for them to call. I wanted confirmation that all was well.

When the nurse told me that they had found cancer in eight of the fourteen sample plugs, I was completely flattened. It was Monday. March was going out like a lamb.

Birds sang merrily. The breeze buffeted me like a late April afternoon in Bermuda, sweet and soft and fragrant. The sky was blue. And all I could hear in my head was, "Oh my God, I am going to die."

If you don't have a similar reaction, I'll be worried about you. It will and should feel like a freight train knocking you down. The train's cars will pummel you again and again, in lightning succession, and when the train passes, you'll feel you have been mortally hit but can still hear your own voice.

This, as they say, is the call to action.

I immediately called my two closest friends, blurting the news to sympathetic ears and mercifully already feeling tears form. I was frantic and could barely catch my breath. Moreover, I could hardly comprehend the words coming out of my own mouth.

Here's the drill. Tell every single person you know. This will trigger a remarkable watershed. Everyone knows someone who has gone through, or is going through, this same thing - this terrifying rite of passage for one out of six men, by the time they are seventy years old.

Stay on the phone constantly. It is not only a lifeline of loving support, but more importantly it produces a magical team of strangers who will, for the critical stages of the ensuing journey, be your warrior brothers and sisters.

Within hours of the diagnosis, I was in touch with five more friends - some of them from the childhood gang who reappeared in the past two months - who put me in touch with five men who had been through this or were facing imminent surgery or treatment. Friends of friends. But initially total strangers who dropped everything they were doing to help another total stranger.

Write everything down. Their phone contacts, their email addresses, their doctors, their hospitals, their reactions, anxieties, fears. The questions they had when diagnosed. The options of treatments. Write everything down because, above all, it will make things real and help stabilize you, almost instantly. You won't feel happy, but you will feel relieved with the confirmation that this happens to others, that you are not alone, and that you will get through it.

By having to gather information and opinions and support, you will gather your breath and start breathing again. And as my closest friend and advisor says, "Breathing is permitted."

Grab everyone you can and place them on all sides of you. It reminds me of an acting exercise called "Trust". One person stands at the center of a group of people who closely encircle him. He places his hands down at his sides, rigidly, and closes his eyes - falls one way or the other - is caught and returned upright to fall in another direction and be caught again. This happens over and over until what starts out as anxiety suddenly turns into a kind of blissful acceptance that everything will be supported and will be all right. This can be done figuratively or, better yet, literally, if you can gather eight or ten friends together. I cannot recommend it more highly. It is tangible, physical proof that you are never alone. Never.

One of the childhood friends I emailed replied within three minutes saying, "Oh, but, Jamie, this is the most treatable and curable of all cancers. And the technology is nothing short of stunning."

Another friend, who I turned to within five minutes of the diagnosis, calmed me down by actually making me laugh. "Hey, Brother! We're all going to get cancer. This is the kind we want!" It seemed way too harsh, in the moment, but it did throw me off guard, make me laugh, and it is true - and critical to keep in mind. Prostate disease is NOT a death sentence. I repeat, it is not a death sentence. It is a passage. Some have even gone so far as calling it "the middle-aged man's measles."

A classmate cousin emailed me, a moment later, to "Fight this with everything you've got. Everything."

And so you can. And so you do.

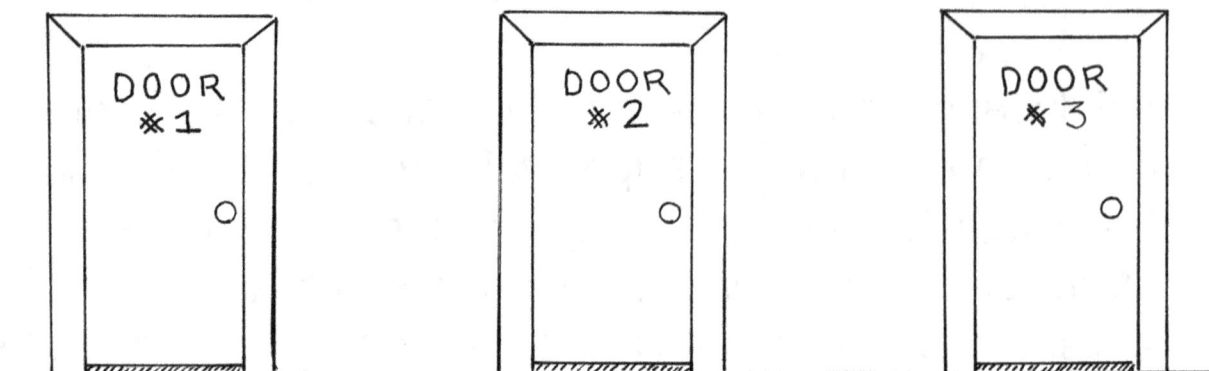

Chapter 6

<u>CHOOSING A COURSE OF TREATMENT</u>

The days couldn't go by quickly enough until I returned to see the biopsy doctor and his associate. Two female friends accompanied me. Nurturing and clear-headed. Even if you have a spouse or life partner, take another friend along if you can. You will hear everything you are told, but will likely not retain nor make sense out of half of it. It's simply that overwhelming to process. Your friends will ask questions you hadn't thought of, and they will take notes. Your job is to ask whatever questions you have, but mainly to breathe and be present in the moment with the experts.

It was explained to us that five of the eight samples which showed disease were very slow growing. The other three, though, were of the type that is very aggressive. I didn't know there were two types of prostate cancer. About 80% is slow-growing, and 20% is aggressive. The slow-growing disease can be left alone and monitored and likely not be at all a problem. But the aggressive type is what kills.

Let me stop here, a second, and reiterate that PSA tests are not just for men over fifty anymore. As I said earlier, there was a 'lad' in my group who was thirty-eight years old. Now doctors strongly recommend keeping track of PSA numbers, yearly, from age thirty-five on. The test has been wrongly criticized, lately, as unnecessary. This is dangerous and, I feel, negligent. Yes, it's an imperfect test. But it's all we have at the moment, and it saves lives. It saved mine. And remember - you don't have to have an entire physical for this. You should also have a ten-second digital exam. That's it. Once a year. Not expensive. Not time-consuming. Start now.

Given my age of fifty-nine, the doctor explained that I was too young a candidate to elect the 'watchful wait' option. If I were ten or fifteen years older, that would be a viable option. But given my age, and considering that some of the samples showed very aggressive disease, he recommended a plan of action.

My choices, then, were radiation or complete removal - either conventionally or robotically. Radiation can involve the implantation of gold seeds in the gland that will facilitate pinpointing the radiation treatment. This, though, means eight to ten weeks, five days a week for about fifteen minutes. The sheer thought of that schedule made my stomach turn - let alone my wallet. It would mean I would have to move to New York City for two months, or commute five days a week, taking up the entire day traveling there and back. Some may feel comfortable having radiation treatments locally. Deep in the country, with limited choices, I did not.

Surgery was then explained in detail. The conventional surgery leaves you with a Caesarian scar from north to south and a long recovery. Robotic da Vinci surgery leaves you with five three-quarter inch scars, one inch-and-a-half scar, and a speedy recovery. So speedy, in fact, that you are released the next morning (pending any complications) with only a one-night hospital stay.

The down side to each: while robotic prostatectomy is currently state-of-the-art, it is still complete removal and the effects can be temporary or long-term incontinence and/or impotence. For most men, these two very important issues will be temporary. And the trade-off is that you are still on the planet to grow older and enjoy your friends and irritate others, or the converse. But it is a scary prospect to be losing one's ability to have an erection. And almost worse - at least for me - was the thought of having to spend the rest of my years on this wondrous planet in diapers.

Radiation, it was explained, can be very effective initially - for a year or so - but disease can recur, and must be treated with either more radiation and/or chemotherapy. Surgical removal, on the other hand, can cause more complications up front, which generally, gradually resolve themselves over time and with therapeutic 'tools'.

I was lastly told that with radiation, if disease does recur, ensuing surgery is a less effective option because the radiation has scarred the area and makes clean removal very difficult.

Between this news and the thought of my body being bombarded by radiation, my choice was absolutely easy. "Take it the Hell Out!"

For many, many men this will be a very fraught decision - whether to keep the prostate or not. For me, I had no hesitation. I would rather stay on Mother Earth longer, with the possibility of incontinence and lack of erections, than not. There is a small risk that one or the other or both conditions will be permanent - this depends on how much cutting the surgeon needs to do. In my case, I was told the risk was low.

But many men will find it formidable to wrap their minds around the possible reality of not ever having an erection again - or whenever they feel like it. There are however, treatments that can be used to achieve an erection - pumps and injections - that for most, work quite well. More about these later.

The Wizard of the Emerald City, in the land of Oz, wisely once said, "Remember, my sentimental friend, that a heart is not judged by how much you love, but by how much you are loved by others."

Similarly, my sentimental reader, there is infinitely more to being a man than your erection.

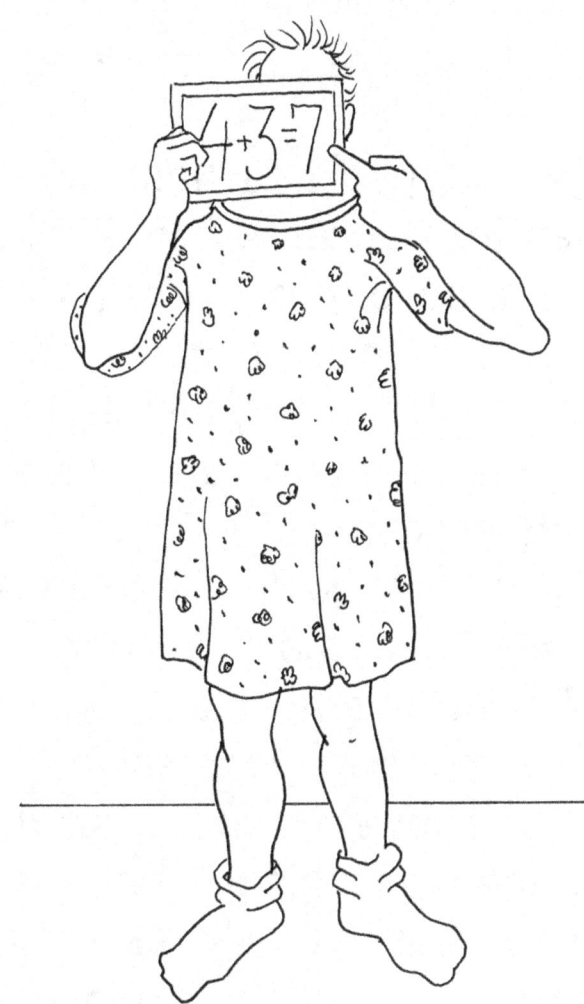

Chapter 7

<u>YOUR</u>
<u>GLEASON SCORE</u>

The Gleason score was invented in 1966 by Dr. Donald Gleason, a pathologist. He based the score on information derived from studies of the biopsies of nearly 3,000 patients who had been diagnosed with prostate cancer. Pathologists worldwide rely on the Gleason score. The score provides an effective measurement that helps your doctor determine how severe your prostate disease is, based on the appearance of the cancer cells when viewed under a microscope. All cancer looks abnormal to a pathologist, but low-grade cancers have cells that often look similar to healthy cells from the land or organ that has been affected by the cancer. But when the cancer is aggressive, the cells look less and less like normal prostate cells (or any other kind of cells).

Pathologists find the Gleason grading system to be very reliable. For example, if the Gleason score indicates that the cancer is an intermediate-risk type of cancer (a Gleason score of 7), it nearly always is an intermediate risk. As a result, doctors can make predictions from Gleason grades. The more distorted and aggressive the cancer looks, the higher the Gleason grade - and the more the cancer behaves aggressively in the body.

The lowest number on the Gleason grade scale is 1, and the highest is 5. This sounds like a contradiction to the above, but actually two Gleason grade numbers are determined and then added up to get the final Gleason score.

Here's how it works: The pathologist looks at the biopsied tissue samples through a microscope to determine where the cancer is the most prominent (the primary grade) and then where it's next most prominent (the secondary grade). Next, he or she assigns a score from 1 to 5 to each area: one score for the primary grade and one score for the secondary grade. The Gleason score is the sum of the primary and secondary grades. As a result, the total score can be anything from a 2 (1 + 1) to a 10 (5 + 5).

The lower the score, the better. A combined Gleason score of 10 is very bad (although there are still many treatments that doctors can offer men with high Gleason scores). Here's how the scores break down:

Scores from 2 to 4 are very low on the cancer aggression scale.

Scores from 5 to 6 are mildly aggressive.

Scores of 7 to 8 indicate that the cancer is moderately aggressive.

Scores from 8 to 10 indicate that the cancer is highly aggressive.

A tricky little feature of the Gleason score for you to keep in mind: The Gleason score usually is reported with the primary cancer number given first, and the secondary cancer number reported second. For example, if Sam's Gleason score is reported as a 4 + 3 = 7, the primary cancer number is a 4, and the secondary cancer number is a 3. Add them up, and they equal a total Gleason score of 7. But remember, not all Gleason scores are equal.

It may sound strange, but if the pathologist classifies Evan with Gleason scale numbers of 3 and 4, which gives him a Gleason total score of 7, Evan is actually in a little better shape, cancer-wise, than Sam. Here's why. When the primary grade (the first number) is 3, it means that the cancer has not advanced as far with cellular deterioration as cancer with a primary grade of 4 (such as is the case with Sam's score). Even though their total scores still equal 7, Sam's and Evan's Gleason scores aren't exactly the same.

So if you want to know the real deal on your Gleason score, get a breakdown of the two numbers that comprise the score. Ask your doctor for your Gleason score, starting with the primary grade first, followed by the secondary grade, and then the total.

The Gleason score from the prostate biopsy (which is just a few slivers of tissue from the cancer) may not be exactly the same as the score the pathologist calculates after surgery, when he or she is able to look at all the cancer in the entire, removed gland. Sometimes the score goes up a little, and sometimes it goes down a little.

The Gleason Score is an important prostate cancer diagnostic tool. It gives you an idea of your prognosis. Then, too, understanding it helps you make an informed decision when it comes to selecting the best treatment options in your situation.

My scores pre-surgery and post-surgery were 3 plus 4, total 7. Dominant nodule was 3 + 4, with a Comprehensive Secondary report of 3 + 3.

At this point, I knew I should have tried to apply myself harder solving those grade school math problems which troublingly started with, "If an apple, an orange, and a pomegranate leave Baltimore at one o'clock, two o'clock and three o'clock, respectively, traveling at the rate of forty-seven miles an hour..."

Seriously - who'd of thought you would ever need to understand this in the real world? And, much more to the point, who authorized fruits to drive?

My biopsy doctor concurred with my desire to have the prostate removed, and gave me the name of a surgeon, in his group, who did robotics. When I read the surgeon's bio, in the office pamphlet, I was somewhat underwhelmed that he had performed over 360 of the procedures.

Just then, the phone rang and one of my closest friends said, "You should talk to Vance. He had robotic prostate removal two years ago." This would be advice from someone geographically close, as all the others were at least three hours away. So I telephoned Vance.

Without hesitation, he said, "I want you to see my surgeon in New York City." After speaking for an hour or so,

I looked up his surgeon on the Internet. His bio stated that he had done, at that time, over 3,600 procedures. I decided that if I liked him, after a consultation, I would certainly go with someone who has done ten times as many of these surgeries as the other fellow.

Before I made the appointment I checked with my insurance group to confirm that I had coverage for the surgery. I did, and it was a great relief, of course. Vance added that I might get bills, subsequent to the surgery, for astronomical amounts, before the hospital and insurance carrier come to an agreement for payment.

I did not receive these, thankfully, but was glad that I was warned ahead of time.

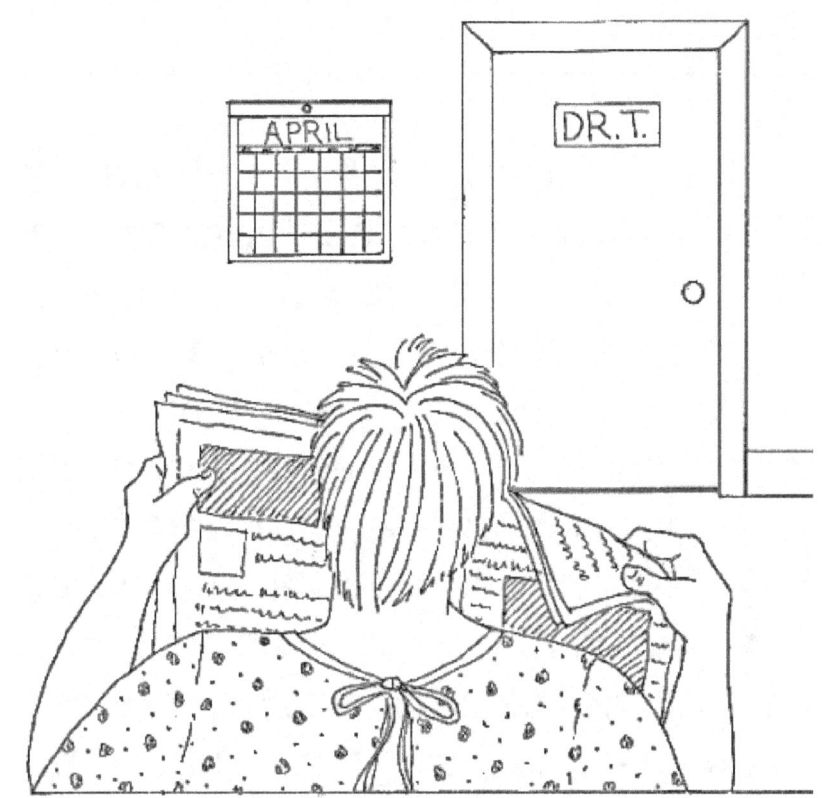

Chapter 8

THE
CONSULTATION

Not only consult with as many doctors as you can (be aware that most insurances allow coverage for a second and a third opinion), but do it as quickly as possible, whatever your Gleason score is at the time.

And again, take at least one extra set of ears. I took two old friends, males, who have each known me for more than thirty years.

My appointment with Doctor T. took place April 23rd - slightly less than four weeks after the biopsy results. All this couldn't have happened quickly enough for me. Bob met me in the hospital's lobby, and we were subsequently joined by Joe upstairs in the doctor's reception room.

The anxiety of the diagnosis, coupled with anxiety over how to choose a surgeon, was a heavy weight to bear. I was very much hoping that I would be comfortable with Doctor T. I had seen a video on his website, where he was shown consulting with a man and his wife. Pre-surgery. Surgery. Then results - and a sigh of relief happy ending. He came across as very warm and caring and confident. What struck me the most was his statement that every time he has to share post-surgery results with a patient, he feels every bit as anxious as the patient does. *This is the guy for me,* I told myself.

After having my vitals taken by Doctor T.'s two assistants, I was told that my blood pressure was a little elevated.

"Oh, really? It couldn't have anything to do with me just BEING here, could it!?" I blathered. They said this was common, but they like to have a baseline on you for each visit. After a bit, Bob, Joe, and I were shown into an examination room, greeted by Doctor T.'s physician assistant. She was lovely and warmly reassuring. She told us what the doctor would be addressing, went over the results of the biopsy briefly, and asked us if we had any questions.

I felt myself start to go on auto-pilot.

The hardest thing about consulting with your surgeon, the first time, is walking out your front door. Once you're actually in the doctor's office, your task really is to let the positive and highly-trained energies take over. This is a blessing because, in my case, she mentioned they were somewhat concerned about the disease being wholly contained in the gland. And that the doctor would be ordering a bone scan.

She left the room, and my heart sunk. The biopsy doctor had told me that they would not need a bone scan. Joe saw this shadowing me, stood up and said, "I think someone needs a hug." Some tears quickly spilled onto his shoulder, which was of great comfort and help. It allowed me to better focus on Doctor T., who knocked on the door shortly thereafter.

I am very lucky to have had a doctor with such grace and warmth. The moment he stepped into the room, the energy palpably shifted.

After shaking everyone's hand, he sat down and we made some small talk. I mentioned that I'd been to his website, and had seen he was a hiker and photography enthusiast. We chatted about my eight-year house renovation, all done myself, how I was rescued by a stray dog six years earlier, and about his dog and such.

Then he rolled his stool nearer to me, and said, "Tell me where you are."

My chin quavering, I replied that I was scared to death.

"Good," he said. "That is energy. Strong energy. And together, we are going to take that energy and turn it into beating this and having a victory."

It wasn't New Age. It wasn't Pollyanna. It wasn't frightening. It simply felt like I was being presented with a path through and out of a very dense, dark forest.

Not every doctor will be as blessed with this aura, as Doctor T. is, but it is important to try as hard as you can to find a surgeon you feel you can trust. Ideally there should be a coin that drops when you've found the right one. Part of this is the person you've found, but it is as much you allowing yourself to be vulnerable enough to need the support.

We talked about details of the surgical procedure. Of the amount and location of the disease within the prostate gland. He used the metaphor of an orange as the gland, saying that they ideally want the disease within the 'pulp' of the orange, and not in the 'skin' of the fruit. I asked about possible side effects and how to treat them. He spoke of the risks involved in major surgery. I asked that, since this is a teaching hospital, would he be the one at the console directing the robot, or would it be someone else? He smiled and gave me his word that he would be the only one at the console. We went over the risks involved, which he stated constituted less than 5% all put together.

Bob and Joe had questions, and made notes, and after about forty-five minutes of discussion, Doctor T. asked me if there was anything else I needed to know from him. There had not been a moment where we felt that he was watching his watch. I felt that if I'd had another thirty minutes of questions, he would have gladly afforded us the time to answer. This was very unusual, especially for a doctor in a major city.

I shook my head that I thought our questions were finished, and then he said, "I want you to promise me something." I nodded hesitatingly. He rolled his stool close to me, taking one of my hands in both of his. "Promise me that the night before surgery, you'll email me and tell me everything we talked about today - tell me of your dog, and the house renovation journey, and my hiking and photography - everything. The morning of surgery, I will read that email and be refreshed and ready to go to work with you." And he handed me his card. "Will you promise me this?"

My eyes were welling up as I shook his hand, "Yes."

Then he added, "This is not just my job. It is my absolute reward."

He exited the room with a beaming smile, leaving behind three grown men absolutely brimming with emotion, wonderment and gratitude that someone could be so generous and sensitive. That he could come into a room with three strangers, ask me where I am, acknowledge my fear, ask me if he could join me in that feeling, and then guide me out of that place in solid partnership with him.

Not everyone will be as fortunate as I was in being referred to this gentle man. Perhaps the universe presented him to me because it knows what a wimp I am when it comes to this sort of thing. But whichever surgeon you choose, feel as strongly as you can about that person, for you must surrender yourself to him or her - completely. And when you do, you will have a tremendous load off your shoulders.

That night, I sent him an email of thanks and a picture of Anio, the Golden Retriever, smiling in the spring breeze.

I closed it with, "Erections be Damned! Cut Away!"

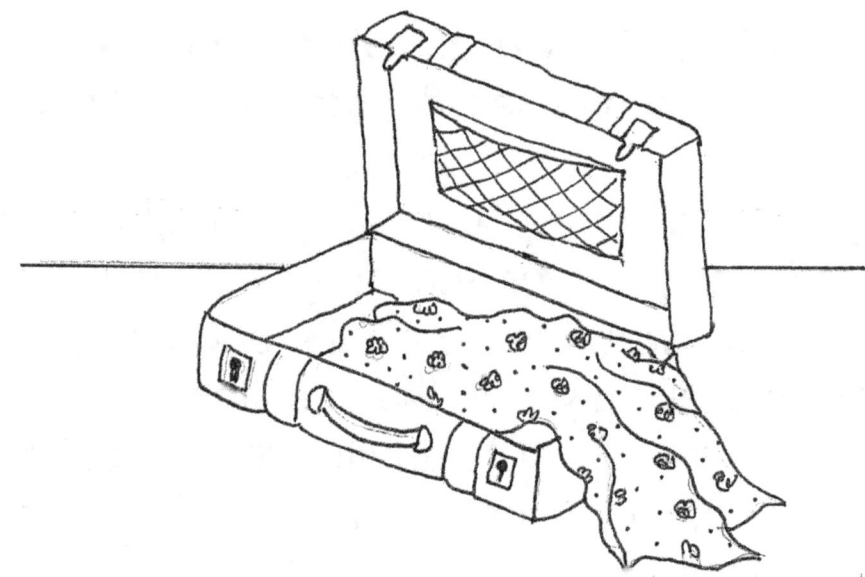

Chapter 9

PREPARING
FOR SURGERY

The days were agonizingly long waiting for a surgery date. The rule of thumb is that there must be eight weeks of healing from the biopsy before surgery. That put me at the third week of May, at the earliest. After a bit of a tussle with the scheduling department, I finally got the date of May 25th. Twenty minutes later, my phone rang.

It was one of the childhood friends who had emailed earlier to say that she had been told my news by another classmate, and that she would be ringing me as soon as she got home from work and got a glass of wine under her belt.

"When did we last talk?" Debbie asked me.

By hit or miss deduction, we figured out that it had been at least 27 years. We did a quick catch-up of geographies and such, and then she asked what hospital I was going to for the surgery. After I told her, her next question was the hospital's address in NYC. Then came, "Who's taking you to the hospital?"

I replied that I had literally just gotten the appointment twenty minutes earlier. I was no where near addressing who would take me.

She took a sip of her wine and said, "Okay, here's what's going to happen. You're going to take the train down to the city the afternoon before. I'm going to take a few days off from work and take the train from Delaware. You'll come to my daughter Emily's apartment at 81st and Second. We'll feed you dinner and put you to bed in her room. She and I can sleep on the fold-out couch. I'll wake you up and walk you to the hospital and check you in. Then I'll be in the recovery room with you, settle you into your room, and drag your sorry, white ass where you need to go the next day."

Tears coursed down my cheeks. "Are you there?" she asked.

"I'm here, I was just...I'm crying."

"Oh, hell, don't do that. Now let me give you Emily's address and phone number."

Another weight, that I'd only borne for twenty minutes, was off my shoulders. I didn't even have the time to contemplate this one. What I had needed was someone to step in and take charge. And she did. And I will never, never forget how much that helped me move forward. Bless Girl Power for taking over...

Once you have a date for surgery, you will feel enormously better. You'll know action is underway. There will be a game plan. There will be results, and most likely they will be in your favor.

SIDE NOTE: Facing the cessation of producing semen, men often elect to have some of their semen frozen. I did not, but consult with your doctor if you do.

For at least three weeks before surgery you should be exercising. Walking is best because not only is it low-impact and good cardio, but it gets blood circulating where you need it most. The more blood flow in your southern regions, the better healing after surgery. Losing a little weight is always desirable, but it is mainly the movement and circulation.

I walked three miles a day at a local school's track. I found it safer than walking our country roads, because I could practically close my eyes and Zen out on the safe track. No traffic. No stumbling over potholes. No attacks by killer squirrels or crazed cyclists. Get some earphones and some tunes and get moving. Not only is it important for your surgery and recovery, it is a meditative time each day that will go a long way in freeing you from anxiety.

At first, the expanse of track looked endlessly long. I could barely imagine going around it once, let alone twelve times. I started to feel sorry for myself. Why was this happening to me? As I continued to whimper, a hand slapped my face. My own. The answer came back, because it has. And because it happens to millions of men. So you realign your thinking and watch one foot step in front of the other. I shifted my focus from the expanse of track to the two sneakers I looked down upon. If I could do this - taking one step at a time - I could do today. If I could do today, rather than taking on the whole impending journey, I could get through the surgery and recovery.

Just tell yourself you can do it. You may find yourself chanting softly or shouting loudly - or everything in between - but keep reassuring yourself.

One morning, in the shower, I heard myself say, "All the strength I need, I already have." To my recollection, I had never heard this nor read it anywhere before. It simply 'arrived'. (Aren't long hot showers miracles, sometimes?) Over the ensuing months, it would become an oft-employed, Mobius-like sentence that never ended. My gift from Hattie McDaniel to you.

I also spent regular time on my rowing machine - especially when it was too hot to do the three miles of walking. With a flat screen television on the wall in front of me, I discovered that I actually enjoyed watching *The Waltons* on reruns each afternoon at five. It's a show I dismissed as a young adult, but I found the hour long program fit the bill perfectly. It was homey and inspiring and it often made me cry.

And besides exercising, crying is the best thing you can do. It can get rid of stress and anxiety - maybe only for a little bit, but everything you can do to be good to yourself you must do. I found screaming at the top or bottom of my lungs very helpful, also. You'll likely be carrying around more anger than you've ever had, and bellowing - in a safe environment - is fantastically helpful. It's a form of fighting back, of affirming that you are going to get through this. Just warn the neighbors and your family, or use a big pillow.

To prepare your muscles for regaining continence as quickly as possible after surgery, Kegel exercises - working out your pubococcygeus muscles (PC) is a tremendous help. It will also give you additional distraction and a regimen while waiting for surgery. And if you can pronounce it correctly - on the first try - I'll send you a dinner for two in Vegas.

'Pubococcygeus', not 'Kegel', wise guy....

PC muscles control the flow of semen and urine. Semen, following your prostatectomy as I've mentioned, is not something you will have to control. There will be none. But there will be urine. And continence is something you will desire more than anything. The great thing about Kegel exercises is that you can do them anywhere, anytime - and no one even has to know you're doing them.

The easiest way to locate your PC muscles is to - without your hands - stop your flow of urine when urinating. Another way to isolate them is to put your finger inside your anus; when you contract the right muscles, your anus and sphincter muscles will tighten. Some describe it as contracting to raise their testicles. However you decide to find them, once they are found you need to practice feeling exactly where they're located because it is easy to overcompensate for weak PC muscles by using the abdominals, buttocks or thighs. These must all stay relaxed when doing Kegels. It is a very small and isolated area - in fact, at first, it may feel like you're not doing anything. But as you practice, you will notice the subtle difference between doing them well, and cheating with abdominals and such.

Your doctor will recommend a regimen to start practicing at least three weeks prior to surgery. These exercises can be done almost anywhere, but I found that sitting on the couch was the most comfortable. You just don't want to be multi-tasking. Do NOT do them while driving. Like any good exercise, you want to be focused - especially in the beginning. That said, don't overdo them. As with any other muscle you're working out, you need to give it time to heal between sessions.

There are a variety of sequences you can go through: contract the muscle for a count of ten, then relax for a count of ten. Do ten sets of these, then take a break. Or you can do ten sets of twenty and twenty. Any combinations are fine as long as you alternate back and forth. Finish up by holding the contraction for a full minute, or even two. You can also do quick back and forths in rapid succession.

Be aware of what you are doing, and if you feel like you are contracting any other muscles (mainly abdominals and thighs), then you need to relax and start again. Take your time. It will pay off in the end...I mean, afterwards. Sorry...

Your doctor will also instruct you not to take any blood-thinning medications or supplements for ten days prior to surgery. No aspirin. No fish oil, et cetera. The last thing you want when having major surgery is 'thinned' blood. Makes sense, right?

Two weeks before surgery, you'll likely have a pre-op bone scan and a CAT scan, as well as an MRI of your prostate. My two scans were done locally. I was anticipating feeling claustrophobic, but greatly relieved to find that both were the open type of scan - not in the least uncomfortable. Short and sweet. Then, of course, another distressing wait for results. Oh, joy...

I, of course, was fearing the worst - that the disease had spread to other parts of my body. My local doctor reassured me that it was standard hospital practice to get a baseline of everything before surgery. This helped a bit as the days went by. Six days later, Kristie read me the results over the phone.

Three of the sweetest words I would hear throughout this entire journey were: "All organs unremarkable."

Then she added, somewhat concernedly, "You know, you have two little gallstones and a fractured right big toe...?"

More phone calls and emails to loved ones reporting another hurdle crossed. I even contemplated whether Doctor T. could remove the gallstones while he was in there. Then I heard Colonel Klink's voice:

"MacKen-ZIE!! Stop being such a cheap bastard!!"

Okay. Now for the MRI.

Your surgeon will order up an MRI of the prostate so that he or she has a topographical map, if you will, of the gland as a guide when doing the surgery. It takes about forty-five minutes from start to finish.

This took place in the city on a Sunday, of all things, which made it pretty low key. Armed with two Ativans in my pocket, on Kristie's recommendation, I arrived at the check-in desk. An old friend, Miles, joined me shortly thereafter, as support and conveyance to the train should I be slightly disoriented following the MRI.

The nurse showed me into a changing room, where I donned the gown that is so very easy to tie in the back. Can't someone design a Velcro closure for these things? Maybe they resist improving on them so they can determine if your Ativans have kicked in yet or not. I remain convinced that no amount of motor skills can conquer the hospital gown on the first attempt.

I emerged to sit in a cubicle until the assistant collected me. Passing a chap sitting in his cubicle, I smiled, and asked how he was doing. He said he'd done this before. I asked if it was claustrophobic. "It's no big deal," he grinned, "It's just like lying in a coffin."

I heard myself laugh as I was cringing inside. Gallows humor was not what I wanted in that moment. But, damn it, it is what you need. And he was trying his best.

Since the area the MRI is scanning is only from the waist down, the good news is that although it is a more conventionally closed machine, your head never goes inside the tight quarters. Although I didn't realize it, my Ativans must have kicked in because I was a little clumsy getting myself situated on the table. Then before I knew it, the young assistant rather rudely shoved a large wand in me. What - no foreplay? I was grateful for the Ativans. She could have warmed the thing up and she could have been more gentle. But after all, she was in there on a Sunday - and perhaps she was having trouble at home with her cable.

Contrary to my expectation, the MRI was actually pretty cool. The technician, on the other side of a glass wall, keeps checking in with you, over a speaker, to see if you're all right. Cautioned that the MRI noise could be hard on the ears, I had brought along good wax earplugs which softened things somewhat. Or maybe it was the Ativans that softened things. All I knew was what started off as sequences of thrumming noises, melted into short symphonies from all over the globe, weaving themselves together in ever changing patterns and rhythms. Classical. African. Asian. Tribal. The Andes. Gregorian chants.

Complex. Quiet. Intricate. It was uplifting. It was celestial. It was fantastic. "God bless modern chemistry," Homer Simpson said, in my head. "God bless us all."

Afterwards, Miles threw me in a taxi headed towards the 125th Street station. Thinking I was on time for the train, he walked me up onto the platform, where we hugged goodbye. "Call me as soon as you get home, okay?" he shouted as he disappeared down the platform, thumbs up, with that great smile of his.

Unfortunately, the train came and went without me and several others. The wrong track number had been posted and announced. I couldn't believe it. I would have to wait an hour and half before another one would arrive. I wanted to be home. I needed to be nestled in my bed with the kids. Liquid massive frustration stung my cheeks.

Many a time I would hear myself repeating a quote from Isak Dinesen: "The cure for anything is salt water - sweat, tears, or the Sea."

If you can work in all three, you'll be way ahead of things - and ready to go.

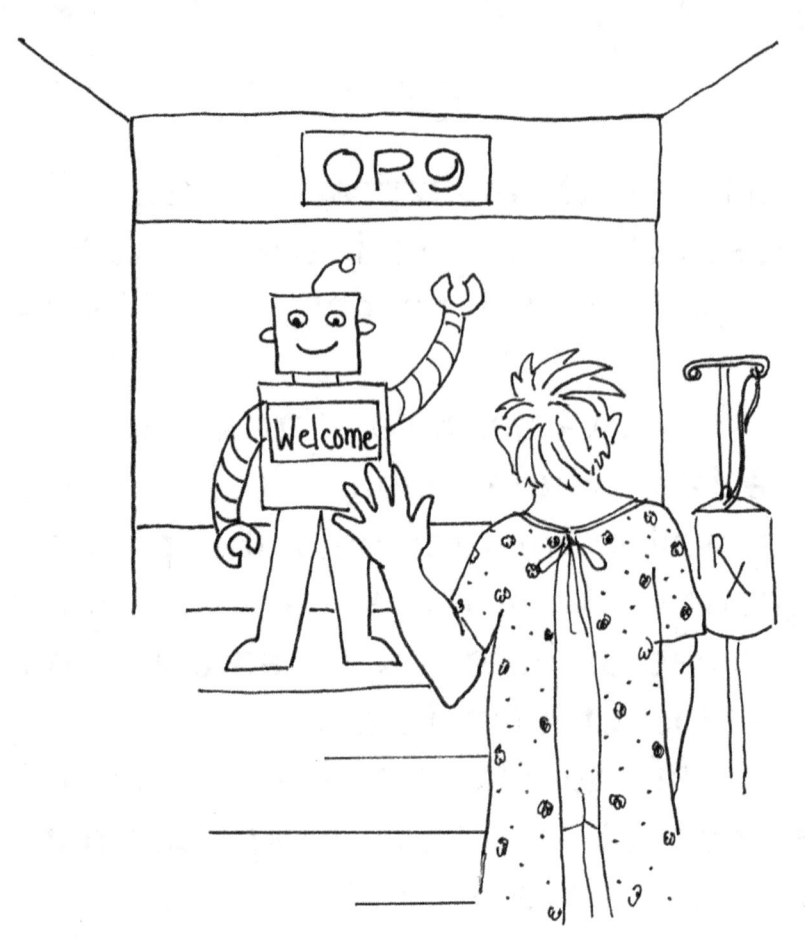

Chapter 10

<u>THE</u>
<u>BIG DAY</u>
<u>ARRIVES</u>

A legal caveat before surgery. If you don't already have one, make sure you have your attorney compose a living will and power of attorney papers, that you sign and have witnessed. The hospital will require it. God forbid anything should go wrong, right? This is so simple and boilerplate - and doing so will not only leave you feeling more secure, it will guarantee you'll come through with flying colors. Your attorney keeps one set. Give the second set to your designated POA, and take the third one to the hospital. They will ask for it when you check in. And, of course, it goes without saying, that you already have a conventional will.

You do, don't you?

Also, make sure you compose a list of names and phone numbers of those who will want to know what your hospital room number and phone number are, and how you're doing. Hand the list to your partner who checks you in.

Depending on where and what time of day you have your surgery, you will either be traveling in the night before or early the morning of. I was scheduled to check in by 8 AM, so I took the train, the afternoon before, heading towards Emily's apartment.

Before I left the house, though, I composed and sent the email I promised I would send.

Dear Doctor T. -

OK. So here it is Tuesday afternoon, and I am getting ready to get on the train to come into the city...to work with you tomorrow mid-morning! As promised, I am writing to recount our meeting four weeks ago.

After greeting me, and my pals Bob and Joe, you asked me what was on my mind. I said I was scared and hadn't breathed in three months other than my morning meditations. You said that is energy, and that we will take that and turn it into beating this and victory. I think you won me over right then and there.

We spoke of my dog, Anio (again pictured here with my face also), and how he was a stray who rescued me six and a half years ago. Simply a miracle and my constant co-pilot. (I tried to get him a seeing eye dog harness, so he could come with me, but they shrewdly found me out.) He will be holding down the fort looking after his two sibling cats, Caleb and Zuzu.

We spoke of your photography and your beloved 13 yr. old lab and hiking. You explained the complications and risks, and assured me that only you will be at the console for the surgery. We spoke of the orange peel and pulp - a great metaphor. And we are hopeful that all is contained. We spoke of my eight year journey transforming the house, here in Taconic, Connecticut - doing all the demolition myself and 85% of the work reconstructing, and how much I enjoy that. (Here're before and after pics.)

I said how much it moved me that your video blog showed you every bit as worried as your patients each time you open the chart containing their results, and that that's what led me to your door. Your open heart.

That you would come in, ask me where I am, acknowledge my feelings and take my hand to bring me out of fear and into partnership with you is a remarkable, remarkable gift for which I am ineffably grateful. I hope I'll see you or hear your voice before - I'll be wearing glasses I had made up because the contact lens will be out, of course. If not, I look forward to seeing you in recovery. Heartfelt thanks - I feel calmer for having written this.

Jamie MacKenzie

A supportive neighbor delivered me to the train station. They and others would be looking after Anio and the cats the next couple of days. All I could repeat to myself, sitting on the train, was *I can do this. I can do this.* Three stops on, I looked up and saw a familiar face. An actor friend, who has a place nearby.

"Bobby!" I hugged him for dear life. He warmly greeted me and within about ten seconds, I told him I was on the way to surgery the next morning. He must have seen the desperation in my eyes, and we sat together for the rest of the hour and a half trip into town. Some really smart angel tossed him in front of me at precisely the moment I needed him. And although it sounds too pat, if you breathe and chant whatever you choose to chant, or pray to whomever you choose to pray - and let go - damnation if someone won't find you. Let them.

Bobby got me all the way into town and we parted with renewed email addresses and phone contacts. Hugging him goodbye, I was off into a taxi to Emily's, where I was met by a face I hadn't seen in almost forty years. Debbie was waiting in the hallway for my elevator. We held each other's faces in our hands and stared through the years of lives led, all the way back to the eyes of four-year old playmates. It was mutual, instant adoration. When Emily opened the door, it was like looking at her mother thirty years ago - so similar were they. So I had this wonderful blend of old and new, trading places, melding into double the joy.

We recounted the years over a light dinner - I being restricted to clear broth only since midnight the night before. After much laughter and blessed distraction, I was off to bed - taking the half a Viagra Doctor T. ordered.

Screeching Halt. Did you say, *Viagra*?!

Yep. Viagra.

WHAT!!!? Hold on! One last fling before saying adios to Mr. Prostate? No. Actually it makes perfect sense. Since erectile dysfunction medication promotes blood flow in the Land Down Under, your doctor wants you to have as much circulation in your pelvic area as possible prior to surgery the next morning. A couple of Ativans took the edge off my anxiety and I was finally able to fall asleep. It was odd being back in the city, hearing the noises which were so familiar from more than fourteen years ago - the hum of air-conditioners, the squeal of sirens, the cooing of pigeons. I ached for the present-day familiar: the closeness of Anio, the Golden Retriever and Caleb and Zuzu, the cats, on the bed with me. But I had two fantastic, two-legged angels on the other side of the door, who were doing everything they could to watch over me.

6 AM. I was already awake when Debbie knocked on the door, and before I knew it, she and I were walking hand in hand down Second Avenue towards the hospital. I kept saying how utterly surreal the whole thing was. I think it was for her, as well. And if it's not for you, too - as I mentioned earlier - I'll be worried about you.

Checking into the hospital. You'll be dreading this the most. Who wouldn't? Just breathe deeply and stay on auto-pilot. My attorney passed along an ancient Celtic prayer to repeat out loud. "All shall be well. All shall be well. In all manner of things, all shall be well."

With Debbie at my side, we made our way to the surgery floor at the hospital. Checked in. Greeted warmly. Donned the Great Equalizer - the hospital gown. Had my vitals taken and a light sedative administered through a drip IV. Sat back down in the waiting room with my new skinny friend - not Debbie - the rolling IV tower. And waited.

I found myself studying each of my gowned co-patients. Most were my age. One was startlingly young; the aforementioned thirty-eight year old. Some of us fell into nervous small talk. Some not. I grasped Debbie's hand continually. Fifty-five years ago, we held hands crossing the road to get to the baseball field for our school's annual Field Day. Held hands on the tour of Gettysburg for our history class trip. Held hands parading to the lunch room where we learned the exotic delights of French dressing on iceberg lettuce. And fell asleep holding hands, nestled in our blankets on squares of cool, speckled linoleum. Now we held hands for another sojourn. No time had passed. No time at all.

"Mr. MacKenzie?" the head nurse called.

Before I knew it I was up and handing Debbie my brand new prescription glasses, which were not allowed in the operating room. I hugged her goodbye, she wished me luck and said she'd see me in the recovery room. A nurse accompanied me and my new buddy, the tower, up a small ramp, around a corner and into a room outside the operating room. No rolling gurney. No glaring ceiling fixtures passing overhead like in the movies. I was - I'll admit - a tad disappointed at the decided lack of drama.

And I expected the operating room to be enormous. After all, there needed to be the table, instruments, room for two physician's assistants, two anesthesiologists, two nurses, the console where Doctor T. would direct the robot's movements, the robot, and Doctor T. It was, in fact, surprisingly cozy. I was 'introduced' to the robot, which stood quietly across the room near the console. It was impressive, but not frightening. Streamlined, but also a little goofy - like a large, grey and white, multi-armed Gumby designed by the Bauhaus boys.

"I come as your friend. Do not be afraid - I will heal you, pitiful earthling."

Yeah, you do that, pal. Knock yourself out.

An intern helped me onto the operating table. It was plain and shiny smooth with a small blue foam neck cradle at one end. The room was noticeably cool, and I recalled reading that this was standard procedure which helps to slow the patient's blood flow. The lights were normal - not gauzy, not dimmed.

I detected a Russian accent coming from one of the interns, and asked him where he was from.

"St. Petersburg," he replied. I proudly rattled off some of my only Russian - the beginning of Hamlet's soliloquy.

Either he or the robot, or both, summarily dismissed me. "Pitiful earthling, resistance is futile."

I don't even remember lying down.

Thanks to breakthrough surgical technology, surgeons now widely offer a minimally invasive option for prostatectomies: the da Vinci prostatectomy, number one in the United States. Just imagine major surgery performed through the smallest of incisions. Imagine having the benefits of a definitive treatment but with the potential for significantly less pain, a shorter hospital stay, faster return to normal daily activities - as well as the potential for better clinical outcomes. And it's named after a pretty decent artist.

With prostate cancer treatment, millimeters matter. Nerve fibers and blood vessels attached to the prostate gland must be delicately and precisely separated from the prostate before its removal. Surgeons use the precision, vision and control provided by da Vinci to assist them in removal of the diseased prostate while preserving important nerves and blood vessels.

As I mentioned earlier, the other great concerns for prostate cancer patients are urinary continence and sexual function after treatment. Studies show patients who undergo a da Vinci prostatectomy may experience a faster return of continence following surgery and lower rates of urinary pain than radiation patients. Several studies also show that patients who are potent prior to surgery have experienced a high level of recovery of sexual function (defined as an erection for intercourse) within a year following da Vinci surgery. Talk to your surgeon about reasonable expectations for recovery of sexual function and a rehabilitation program that may include exercises and drug therapy.

It is important to remember that the robot - however intergalactically charming - is not working on you; your surgeon is always in control of every aspect of the surgery with the assistance of the robotic system. Although, you are free to give your robot a name, if you like. Mine was Mr.

Robot. Well, how clever can you expect to be at a moment like this?

The surgeon's team angles the operating table down at your head, so that your internal organs will gravitate north. This, in addition, to blowing carbon dioxide into your abdominal cavity, is what gives the robotic arms room to maneuver around.

Five vertical incisions are made, each about three quarters of an inch, near your left and right hip in the front - two at waist level, two at the pubic level, and one at your left hip. A single, inch-and-a-half long vertical next to your belly-button is made, through which the gland is drawn out upon removal. And yes, it will be in a little plastic bag for retrieval purposes. Not only can the robot make precision cuts, it uses baggies, too. You don't believe me? Watch the videotape.

Shortly before the operation, your anesthesia is administered and you'll go to sleep for the duration of the operation, which typically lasts two to four hours.

During the procedure, the surgeon uses the da Vinci System's laparoscopic surgical instruments and video camera to direct the dissection of the prostate gland and adjacent tissue. If deemed appropriate, the surgeon tries to preserve the nerves attached to the prostate gland. At the end of the surgery, the incisions are closed with sutures or surgical tape.

"Now that that's that, I insist that you call me 'Jamie'. And I'll call you...?"

"Signor da Vinci!!"

"Right! Sir!!"

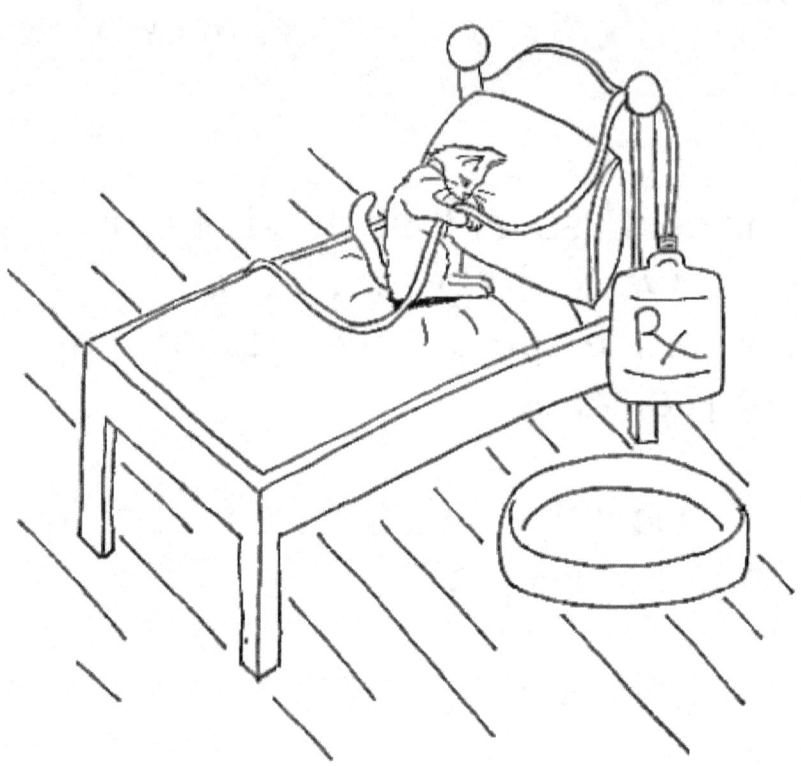

Chapter 11

POST-SURGERY
RECOVERY

You may have wonderful dreams or perhaps terrible nightmares. I had neither.

I blinked. Then wondered who had poured a case of Scotch down my throat and stuffed my mouth with old wool socks. I found this extremely disconcerting. God knows what I must have looked like coming to in the recovery room. Thankfully, they don't videotape it. Most hospitals do record the surgery, but that has to be more interesting than watching someone poorly speaking Klingon while trying to remove stockings from his mouth.

You'll be aware of voices, familiar and unfamiliar. But all of them kindly, in my case. I was not really aware of anything visually - just foggy soft light. And endless, endless socks.

What seemed to be an eternity of clumsy mouth movements was mercifully punctuated by periodic doses of ice chips and morphine. To paraphrase Homer Simpson, "Uhmm...morphine. The cause of, and solution to, all life's problems."

Gradually I became aware of rolling, on a cart, into a brighter room, and being asked to turn over onto my bed. This transition happened quickly and, it seemed, with little effort.

Faces were still unfocused, but voices were becoming more cohesive in their sentence structure. The mouth was still full of laundry, but someone was holding my hand; the gorgeous fifty-nine/four-year old who'd held my face in her hands the afternoon before.

This was early evening, and I recall ringing telephones, though absolutely nothing of any conversation with anyone on the other end of the line, although I was told I did speak something to a few concerned callers. Tylenol with codeine, administered regularly, took care not only of the pain but also put a lovely broad watercolor wash over everything.

Just enjoy it while someone else is paying for it.

A few hours later, after visitors had left, I seemed to be really awake. I mean, five cups of coffee awake - and I don't even drink coffee. I was only allowed a liquid diet - bland 'chicken' broth, and Jell-O that was far too red for its own, or my, good. You could locate it in the dark by its eerie glow. The fact that in four days, I would lose eighteen pounds tells you something about the menu. Same thing, every meal. Every meal.

I was on the liquid diet because Doctor T. found a small section of my colon that had become detached from the wall of my abdomen. He reattached it but wanted to make sure that, for the first few days, no solids were passing through. Much to my chagrin, I watched regular meals being handed out to the others. They didn't look four-star, but they were enviably solid.

I stayed up that first night watching television until around midnight. I was simply too buzzed for some reason. Nurses came and went, checking this and that, and then...oh, did I forget to mention that you'll wake up with a catheter hose coming out of your penis? Sorry about that...

This sort of slipped my mind because you truly are not even aware of it, at first. The meds take care of the intrusive stuff. Up to a point.

There will be a thin, smooth plastic hose, about three feet long, coming out of your urethral opening. It will be connected to a catheter bag on a rolling stand which collects your urine flow. Nothing to worry about, at all. No pain, no discomfort. But a pronounced different vision of the world when you look south. I just don't want you to be totally surprised.

The bag is emptied regularly by helpful nurses, and you will be encouraged to do this yourself as soon as you're able, because you'll likely be the one doing it at home the first week - or at least part of the time.

Urine flows all on its own - you just lie back, smile, and enjoy not having to think about it.

One thing that will become very clear in the first twenty-four hours after surgery, is how completely uninhibited you become about strangers poking and prodding you. You're only wearing a hospital gown anyway. It actually is kind of freeing. Of course, the meds help with any shyness you might have had, but more so, you'll find that you have already done the hardest work - getting yourself in and out of surgery - and you have already given yourself over to those around you who are there to help. Even those people in the kitchen who keep spooning out the Jell-O. Bless their sweet, little radioactive fingers.

The first awareness I had of real pain was the bloating. Everyone goes through this. I am somewhat glad they didn't tell me how bad it can feel. I was warned, but had never experienced anything like this.

Be prepared. Brace yourself. It will feel as if you're repeatedly having a heart attack. For twenty-four to seventy-two hours. Heart attacks. But all you need do is ask your nurse for some meds, and this will help greatly.

During surgery, as I mentioned, the team must blow carbon dioxide into your abdominal cavity, so there is room for the robotic 'hands' to move around and get to where they must. This extra air or gas is not passed in the conventional way - it must be slowly absorbed and then dispersed. This can take up to three days. Which is one of the reasons that they have you up and walking at least a mile the morning after surgery, in most cases. They want the whole system moving and working and eliminating.

It's quite a dreamlike sight, I thought, when I first rolled my tree stand out the door of my room and saw ten or so guys walking up and down the hallway in their wraps and bootied feet. Heaven? Hell? I'll go with Temporary Purgatory. It was uncomfortable, at times painful, but it was also movement towards the future. While it certainly wasn't, by any means, Hell, the absence of an improved hospital gown readily confirmed it wasn't Heaven, either.

The corners of walls are marked, indicating how many portions of miles you have walked. Everyone smiles through their gas pain and nods encouragement to each other. You will find yourself temporarily bonding to one or two of them, and this is very, very helpful. They're going through precisely what you are. Except that they get solid food and I was getting the liquid diet from the Planet Rouge. But I was losing the excess weight I should have lost more of before surgery.

Doctor T. greeted us all that first morning, warmly reassuring each of us that our surgeries had gone well. We flocked around him like little chicks to their mother - eager to please him with our 'odometer' reports, anxious to hear more about our surgeries. This is when he told me about the reattaching of the colon section, and apologized profusely for the liquid diet.

Most of our group went home that afternoon - one day after surgery. I elected to stay one more night, because I didn't want my first night out of the hospital to be three hours away in Connecticut, should any complications occur.

Kind doctor friends had recommended this, reminding me that those are my rights as a patient; to state that I felt I needed another night of care. Remember this, in case you are not feeling totally on your game. It's your right. Speak up.

Before you are released, you will be shown how to change the catheter bag, and also how to empty the port bulb which most men have at their sides. This small flexible bulb - known as a Jackson Pratt drain - is removable for emptying the fluids which are free-roaming. This may start out somewhat rusty but will become clearer as the days proceed. Very easy to handle. It is emptied, then, as it is reconnected to the port on your abdomen, it is squeezed of air so that when connected it acts as a suction to draw excess fluids out.

The Ride Home. A very dear friend dropped everything in his Memorial Day weekend schedule with his wife and kids to come collect me for the two and a half hour drive home. I was anticipating being pretty uncomfortable in Dan's car but, again, the meds will take the edge off this. I think we stopped once - somewhere along the Saw Mill Parkway - to empty the smaller 'walking bag' that was Velcro'd to my thigh, and easily removable.

My four-legged kids were wild with excitement to have me home after almost four days away. Devoted neighbors were rotating schedules for walking and feeding and scooping litter. They will never know how much it meant to me to know that the kids were well looked after.

I slept surprisingly soundly that night, having changed over to the large catheter bag. And I was really looking forward to having my first shower in more than four days.

The next morning, my best friends Cheryl and Dave, dropped by to see how I was making out. I hugged them both, and thanked them endlessly for taking care of things. Then Cheryl said, "Hey, let's see how small your incisions are."

Upon dropping my shorts to the floor (no underwear these days - too warm and way too complicated), Cheryl's exclamation was...how shall I put it? Yeah, 'deafening' will do. Dave groaned almost as loudly. I quickly pulled my shorts up, remembering I wasn't in the hospital any longer. Their reaction, I was later told, was not so much that I was naked, but that they'd never seen a tube coming out of a penis before. Neither had I.

Showering, by the way, is not a big deal. They do not want you taking a bath for the first week, while the catheter is in place. Simply take the bag you're using into the shower with you.

Your incisions will likely be surgical tape - very small and perfectly compatible with water and mild soap. It's very important to note that you should be using an anti-fungal soap. Easy to find at the pharmacy. Gently wash the incision areas and around the drain port at your side, if you have one. You'll likely be given a tube of Lidocaine to swab the head of your penis on a regular basis. Do this after you've dried off from the shower. It will serve to slightly numb the area where the hose inserts, and keep it from getting dry.

Since we're still in the bathroom at this point, you will be using the toilet and hoping for your first bowel movement. Mine took a couple of days because I had been on that all-enticing liquid diet. When it comes to your bowel movements, everything is done the same way you always have. Just be careful not to strain. Let nature take its course.

It's a good idea, if your insurance covers it - and mine fortunately did - to have a visiting nurse (unless you happen to live with one) come and check your incisions, drain port, and catheter during the first week after surgery. My nurses visited three times - before and after the catheter and port removal - and were very helpful and encouraging, making exacting notes and diagrams that were faxed to my doctor.

Once the surgical tape has dissolved on your incisions - usually within a week or so - they may not look perfectly closed. This is where the visiting nurses were important. Some incisions will close more quickly than others. Some men's will close faster than others'. Don't worry. But - do keep them clean with the anti-fungal soap. Do NOT swab them with household rubbing alcohol or hydrogen peroxide. These can burn the tissue and retard the healing. I made this mistake using the peroxide.

Two of my incisions had a small amount of slightly, pale green material in their cavity. I told my local doctor this and she recommended that a swab be taken and sent out to check for infection. Everything came back clear, and I was then ever vigilant about using the soap and letting air get to them.

You may be tempted to use some Band-Aid patches on your incisions, as I did, because three of them are right at your waist line. I found that the patches kept the paper pull-ups from rubbing them. But what really helped close the wounds was air.

So when you can, once you are sitting down for any amount of time, remove the Band-Aids and...welcome the breeze.

Sleep like an Egyptian. Luckily, you'll find your body knows precisely what to do when faced with some extra equipment around your waist - like a catheter. Make certain your large catheter bag is on the floor - not on the bed. It has to be below you for gravity to do its job. Lie on your back, get a couple of extra pillows to buttress you on either side, and you'll find you'll adopt the mummy repose easily. You may still be on pain killers, too. I stopped mine four days after surgery. Sleeping on your side works, also, though best to face the edge of the bed so you don't get tangled up with your catheter. And remember, you don't have to get up to pee in the middle of the night! Just enjoy the sleep.

The smaller bag that enables you to roam around untethered to the large overnight bag, as I mentioned, Velcros around your thigh. It's usually good for a few hours depending on your fluid intake. It, too, has a stopcock that shuts off the flow. Take it off your thigh and empty it out, reconnect, and you're good to go. It is not intrusive, and is perfectly comfortable. And, it's only for a few more days. If you're planning on wearing hot pants, you may want to reconsider.

VERY IMPORTANT: A note about the after-effects of anesthesia. During the first three weeks after surgery, there were times when I suddenly felt frantic - as if something dark was about to pounce on me. It wasn't depression - just a manic, frantic panic - better known as MFP (my expression). It would come and go unannounced, never staying more than an hour or so. When I mentioned this to a close family friend, on the phone from France, he immediately replied, "Well, of course you are feeling zees way, my brother. You must remember you had zree hours of poison in you!"

Prior to this surgery, I'd only had ether for a tonsillectomy (age 5), and a sedative for a colonoscopy - so I was totally unprepared for the psychological and physical havoc prolonged anesthesia can wreak on one's entire system.

Ask your doctor about this, and don't be surprised if there are some of these bumps after surgery. It can be very dark.

It's normal. And it will fade.

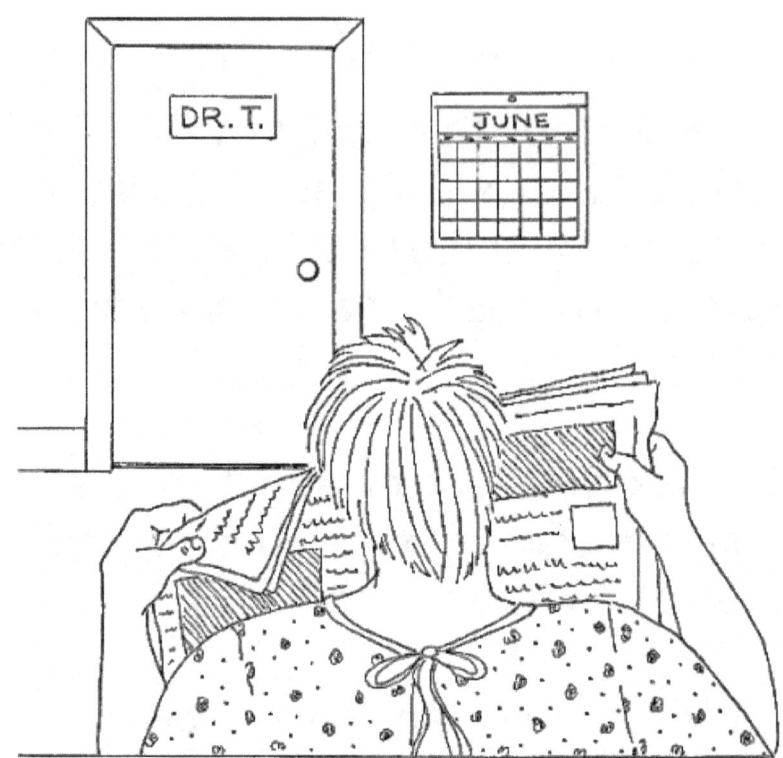

Chapter 12

POST-
SURGERY
RESULTS

I returned to see Doctor T. one week after surgery. Another train trip, another stay at Emily's welcoming apartment to be able to make the 9:30 AM appointment. This visit was to remove the catheter and the drain port line, to check my incisions and, most importantly, to learn more about the pathology work that was done after the surgery. After dinner, we watched three or four episodes of John Cleese's brilliant television series, *Fawlty Towers*. Emily had never seen them before. Highly recommended.

During surgery, samples of the tissues surrounding the prostate gland are taken to make sure that the disease has been contained in the gland itself. These samples are tested on the spot, across the hall while you're on the operating table, in case they deem it necessary to remove more tissue.

This return consultation will be another one of those very anxious moments. Again - take a spouse or friend for support and for another set of ears. My pal, Miles, joined me again for this important step.

One of the many things, as I mentioned earlier, that endeared Doctor T. to me was watching the website video where he held his clipboard and said, "I am just as anxious for every single patient's results as he is himself."

And now it was my turn.

While Miles waited in the reception area, I was taken to an examination room where a nurse would remove the drain port bulb and line, as well as the catheter. On the recommendations of those who'd gone through their catheter removals, I had been preparing myself to have to scream bloody murder. I wasn't thinking at all about the drain port line. So it was truly a surprise when she first yanked the drain line out of my side. I shrieked a string of four-letter words that made the fluorescent lights overhead blink a few times, gathered my breath and promptly apologized. I was also shocked to see how long the line was. Almost six feet! After this, the catheter removal was a cinch. Truly. And remember how lucky you are that the catheter was put in place while you were under anesthesia. Enough said.

Once you are unencumbered, you'll be asked to drink a lot of water. A lot. And wait half an hour or so. This is because they want to see that you can urinate freely. One of the patients from our group was there, also - Scott, the thirty-eight year old - and we quickly began a competition as to who would pee first. After what seemed to be a gallon of water, I had the urge.

Don't be surprised if things feel a little strange. There may be some burning, some hesitation, but most men resume normal urination with a grand, first flow. That said, mine was, directionally, not focused where I anticipated, but it was flowing and for that I was supremely grateful. Kind of like a fire hose out of control, at first - but at least it was putting out the fire.

Once that hurdle had been crossed, and Scott and I had exchanged awards, Miles and I were taken in to see Doctor T. He asked how I was and after a little small talk, looking at my chart, he told me that although he believed all the disease was contained in the removed gland, he found a slightly larger amount of disease than they had expected from the pre-op MRI. My heart began to sink, and I started to float above myself. That's why it's so important to have at least one extra set of ears.

He then said they were going to study the slides more closely to make sure everything was all right. He was warm and positive and told me that he and I would "be dining together in ten years' time."

Although this was encouraging, I guess I had expected him to say everything was great, open a bottle of champagne for us, and start dancing.

I was told that another PSA draw would be taken in six weeks. One more wait. One more hurdle. Well, what else was I doing?

Returning Home. Your first stop, if you haven't already done this, should be to pick up a supply of pull-up diapers from that aisle in the pharmacy/grocery store. These come as full underpants, and also as pads. I started myself off with the underpants, then moved to the pads - which have a peel and stick area to adhere to your underwear. Easily changed during the course of the day. And they work very well.

Now. You will leak or, rather, squirt. Everyone does. When I coughed, I squirted. When I cleared my throat, I squirted. I squirted when I blew my nose, lifted something (which you shouldn't do for the first three weeks, nothing over five pounds), got out of the car - any sort of exertion - especially 'breaking wind'. This is normal, and the protective gear is wonderfully designed to help. That's why you purchased them - to protect your wardrobe in a discreet way. I habitually consume a lot of water - and you will be encouraged to do the same. How much you consume, in the course of a day, will determine how often you'll need to change your gear. At the start, I went through three full pull-ups each day, and one or two overnight. Gradually, over the next two weeks I elected to sleep without the pull-ups. I found them more comfortable for walking than sleeping. But I still occasionally leaked.

A trick I came up with, for sleeping, was to place a folded towel under the sheet at the side edge of the bed, where any leaks might occur (because I generally sleep on my side). This saves the mattress pad and mattress. You may also want to put a square of plastic under the folded towel. Be inventive! And now they have peel and stick pads, mainly designed for bed-wetting children, which will work even better.

I found the most uncomfortable thing about the pull-ups was that my left testicle was extremely sensitive and hurt like the dickens when moved in any direction. I rang the office and was told this was normal but that they also would like an ultrasound done of each testicle. I did this locally and the results were perfectly normal. Many doctors will recommend wearing an athletic supporter the morning after surgery. I found this too uncomfortable, so I may have paid the price for not doing this with the ensuing sensitivity. Check with your doctor.

During the course of surgery, a fair amount of knocking around goes on down there and I may have sustained a strain of sorts which caused the feeling of teen-age 'blue ball'. Ouch! But this subsided as time passed. It took about eight weeks to wear off, about the time that my continence returned.

Six weeks after surgery, I had another PSA test. I think I was the most anxious about this one. I rang Doctor T.'s office to inquire, and was told that the results were 0.064. To me this sounded pretty damn good. The assistant on the other end of the phone agreed, and then added, "We like to see it 0.05 or below." Again my heart sank. How much more of this can I take?

I took a deep breath and asked her if this was cause for concern and she said, "Not at all. It is basically undetectable."

How many friends received my news of "basically undetectable"? Everyone. This was cause for celebration. The relief for me was, need I say, unlimited, and I was also tremendously relieved for all the people who were pulling for me. To give them good news was my greatest hope and accomplishment. Finally. A light at the end of the tunnel. My gift back to them for all their support.

At this point, in late August, life seemed to be getting back to 'relatively normal'.

Unless you're fortunate enough to have yourself a full-time accountant, returning to 'relatively normal' means a lot of paperwork. The bills will seem mountainous at first. Take many deep breaths. Check with your insurance carrier regularly and make certain that it is meeting its responsibilities. If paying the bills is a hardship, turn to the entities sending the bills, and ask them for assistance. They all, generally, have programs to either reduce the amounts owed, or at least spread them out over a reasonable period of time, to make them affordable.

The main thing is this: there is and will be help available. Use it. Because you need to keep focused on your health recovery, not on financial stress.

Another six weeks and another PSA. Thankfully, the results were exactly the same number. What's important here is that your baseline for being cancer-free will be different from the next guy's. I was envious when I heard from Scott that his numbers were 0.008. Extremely low. Don't let this throw you. Everyone tests differently. Keep in mind that one man's cancer-free may be 0.079 and another's may be 0.006. It is the stability of these numbers, over the course of time, that matters.

Mine remain, now in three month intervals of testing, precisely what they had been after surgery. And I am very satisfied with that.

WARNING: Your PSA numbers can differ from one diagnostic facility to another. When my local blood-draw office closed, and I went to another one, my numbers increased two hundredths of a point. The sheer fact that they moved alarmed me. After reporting this to Doctor T.'s office, their immediate question was, "Have you changed diagnostic facilities?" When I confirmed that I had, they replied that it is VERY common for baseline numbers to change from facility to facility. It is consistency - from one ongoing testing lab - that they are looking for.

It is in our nature to do everything we can to regain normalcy. And yet, there will never be normalcy again - or, at least, the illusion of normalcy. This journey redefines everything. And your job, your gift, is to let it.

If the guys you felt so close to, just after your diagnosis - the brother warriors who helped and advised you - disappear or recede, don't be alarmed. I think this is a natural function of the terror stage. After everything has been done and settled, there seems to be a reticence to revisit those harrowing days and conversations, as intimate as they may have been. There comes a type of disassociation from the crisis, which is likely natural for forward movement. Keep in touch if you can. Wish them well. And then let them go to resume their lives and you yours.

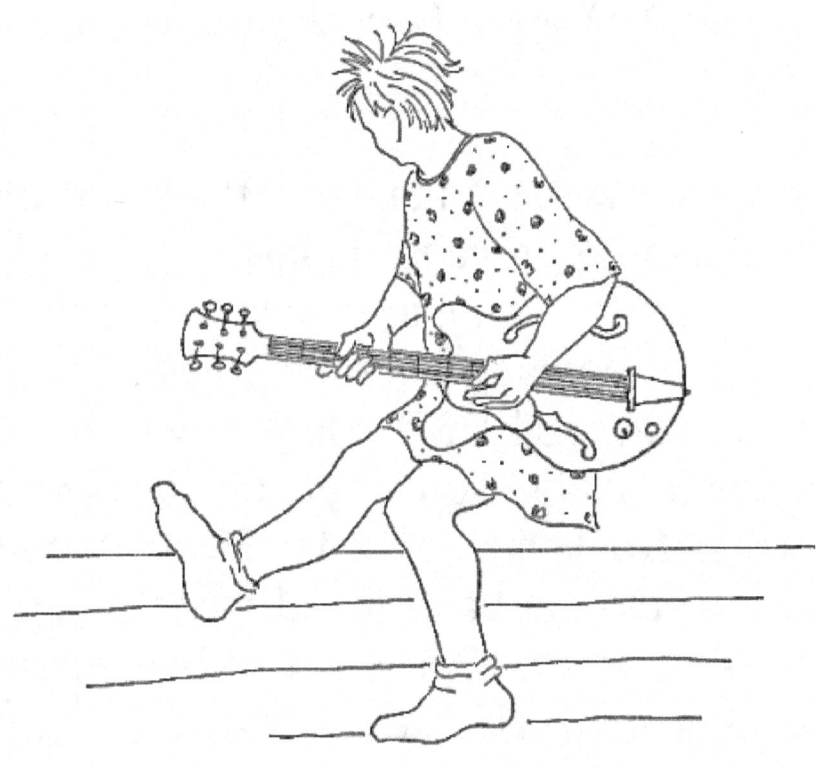

Chapter 13

SEX, DRUGS
& ROCK 'N ROLL

Okay. Continence usually returns sooner than potency, for most men. For the first six weeks - totally absorbed with trying to control my urine flow - I was unconcerned about having an erection, or for that matter even having sex. And because I fell into that three percent of men with side effects from erectile dysfunction drugs, I chose no diarrhea, back aches, or head aches over regaining my erection.

But I did follow doctor's orders and tried 'self-stimulating'. I turned to online erotica (gee, I had that bookmarked...how'd that happen?) and proceeded to attempt to arouse myself. I thought, well, if nothing else happens, I've promoted a little more blood circulation with my doctor-approved frottage.

I started laughing, having grown up with Permanent Catholic Damage - or what we, in the brotherhood and sisterhood, call PCD. Here I was masturbating not at my doctor's suggestion, nay, his insistence! No hair on the palms. No lightning bolts. Even a potential knock at the door would not have fazed me. I heard myself say, in John Cleese's voice, "Sorry, I'm self-stimulating. Doctor's orders, you know. You'll have to wait!" I would not be dissuaded from my mission.

Somewhere into forty-five minutes of absolutely nothing happening down south, I suddenly felt an orgasm coming on. But how could this be, when I didn't have a ghost of an erection? Well, it did - "by golly, Uncle Jed" - it did!

Now, this was not an orgasm on the scale of pre-surgery orgasms - but it was astonishing to be shown that an orgasm can actually take place while being totally flaccid. Clearly, where there's a will, there's a way.

The easy next-joke opportunity is the realization that there is no need for a washcloth as there is, of course, no semen. A cheap joke and a serious subject at the same time. It is completely unfamiliar not to have any ejaculate. It is foreign and made me feel less of who I am or was. I felt a sadness and a lack, but not a regret.

Give yourself time to adjust to this actuality. I still feel odd about it, less so now, but will likely always miss the explosion a full outflow of semen produces - something one has been accustomed to one's entire life. For me, it initially felt quieter, like a 75% orgasm. Though with continued practice, most have been downright terrific, and some even more earth-shaking than before surgery! Everyone is different. Now, a year after surgery, I can say that my orgasms are something to be looked forward to, not something just to be practiced because it's therapeutic. At the end of the day, whatever level of pleasure you experience as orgasming is certainly better than nothing, can be done flaccid or partially flaccid, and you're still here on the planet to have one. Note that you may also involuntarily release some urine prior to, or after, your orgasm. This is perfectly normal.

As time went by, though, and my penis continued to wear the moniker "Mr. Floppy," I started to wonder if an erection, even a partial one, would ever return. I had been cautioned by Doctor T. that this could take as long as a year or more, in some cases - so I was prepared, but hopeful I might beat the odds.

By six months after surgery, and having noticed way too many television commercials for post-prostate surgery vacuum pumps for your penis, I decided to have a talk with Mr. Floppy.

JAMIE: Mr. Floppy?

MR. FLOPPY: (SNORING) ZZZzzzz.....

JAMIE: Mr. Floppy?

MR. FLOPPY: Don't bother me now. I'm resting.

JAMIE: Resting? You're always resting!

MR. FLOPPY: Not always. Remember yesterday...?

JAMIE: Now, let's get serious, M.F. - I want to explore the technology of penile injections to gain an erection.

MR. FLOPPY: YOU...WHAT!!?

JAMIE: Just calm down...

MR. FLOPPY: I am calmed down! I'm flaccid!!
Penile injections!!? Are you out of your mind!? And, yes, 'flaksid' is the preferred pronunciation! Look it up!

JAMIE: Yes, Doctor T.'s office wants all men - as part of their healing and regaining erectile function - to promote circulation on a regular basis.

MR. FLOPPY: You sounded like you were 'circulating' pretty well, yesterday.

JAMIE: That's the point - just because I have an orgasm -

MR. FLOPPY: ...WE have an orgasm...

JAMIE: Yes, WE have an orgasm, doesn't mean that there is healthy blood circulation in you.

MR. FLOPPY: And you're proposing to do what about this, again?

JAMIE: There are vacuum pumps that help, but really only trap blood in you.

MR. FLOPPY: And the alternative is a puh...puh...penile injection?

JAMIE: A penile injection.

MR. FLOPPY: Oh my god - if I could get any limper, I would faint.

JAMIE: Look we have to do this together, as a team, for our health. Now grow up...uhmm, sorry...I didn't mean that. I meant, expand your horizons...no ...It's time to enlarge our knowledge...Oh, shit! I give up!

MR. FLOPPY: No need for potty-mouth, I'm listening...

JAMIE: Injections, with a fluid called TriMix, cause fresh blood to flow to you, which is healthier.

MR. FLOPPY: Okay...

JAMIE: And it barely hurts - one tiny little prick.

MR. FLOPPY: Okay! That does it!! I am so outta here...

JAMIE: Sorry. Sorry! A very small needle. Easily administered. Easily tolerated. No side effects at all. Just a 'stand-up, happy soldier'.

MR. FLOPPY: 'Stand-up', you say? I remember that, I think. Hmmm...and you say it doesn't really hurt?

JAMIE: Barely feel it.

MR. FLOPPY: And it's good for our health...?

JAMIE: Very important for our health.

MR. FLOPPY: Okay. Dial the number and make the appointment. But remember, I'm going with you!

JAMIE: I hoped you'd see it that way.

I felt somewhat ridiculous, and somewhat excited sitting in the waiting room for Doctor T.'s assistant to talk with me about injections, and try one. I had spoken with Adam on the phone, and had a pretty good picture of what to expect. And as I mentioned before, once you go through this journey, you leave all modesty and inhibitions with strangers way behind you.

So, after cordialities, Adam asked me questions about my erections prior to surgery, and what I was experiencing since. He asked about the quality of my orgasms, and I told him that they felt like three quarters of an old orgasm. Sometimes a little less, sometimes more.

He then showed me what is called 'the kit'. This consists of twenty small syringes, antiseptic swabs in individual wrappers, and the medication in a bottle the size that contact lenses used to come in. I would be getting this shipped to me directly from the manufacturer.

ONE NOTE: Penile injections have not, at this writing, been approved by the FDA. They have, though, been shown to be very safe in over eight years of broad use. Each kit costs about eighty dollars, including shipping, and is good for nearly four months of twice-weekly injections. Insurance will not cover it because it is not FDA-approved. But for its contribution towards regaining your erection, its cost is worth it.

Removing the protective sheath from the syringe revealed a very short, fine needle. I gave a half a sigh of relief. After swabbing the rubber drum across the top of the bottle, Adam inserted the needle and showed me how to draw back the proper amount. This will be minimal the first time because they want to see how your penis reacts. Not everyone will need the same amount for an erection that is satisfying. With ensuing injections, you will increase the amount gradually until you feel Mr. Floppy has been, at least temporarily, shown the door.

With a diagram at hand, he showed me that the injection should be located on either side of the penis shaft, about half way down - or in this case, across, since the penis is pulled to one side parallel to the floor.

Then imagine the cylinder of your penis head-on. At three o'clock and nine o'clock, if it were a clock face, are the points to inject. It is also key to make sure the needle is inserted ninety degrees to the skin, and on the same plane - not at an angle going down or going up.

Once the syringe was filled, Adam told me to swab the injection site on my penis.

I dropped my trousers, and Adam showed me where the single injection should be best located. The shaft of the penis should be gently pulled to the left or the right thigh, and held there by one hand or the other. It doesn't make a difference which, for the first time, but it is important to alternate sides as you continue injecting to keep the tissue from unnecessarily scarring. He recommended my left thigh, so I could use the syringe with my dominant right hand.

"Do you think you would like to do this yourself, or would you prefer that I do it?" Adam encouragingly inquired.

Well, I've made it this far, Pilgrim, I thought. What the Hell. "Sure," I replied. So, while pressing my penis against my thigh, I cautiously chose an area as instructed. Adam made a slight adjustment opting for insertion below the major vein that runs along the shaft.

"Okay?" he asked.

"Ready for lift-off," I answered, pushing the needle into Mr. Floppy's side.

Yes, a little sting, but far less than a needle in your arm or buttocks. I did, though, encounter a little resistance. Adam told me to continue pushing until the needle was completely inserted - about three eighths of an inch. He explained that the outside tissue needs to be pushed freely through.

I pushed the plunger all the way down, then retracted the needle.

If you're still with me at this point, it was really nothing. If, on the other hand, you've just keeled over, feel free to reread this when you're back on your feet. I can wait.

"Your call is very important to us. Please hold. (PAUSE).....*Raindrops keep falling on my head, and just like the guy whose feet are too big for his...*" Oh, there you are. Welcome back.

The worst aspect to this, of course, is the sheer thought of doing it. It's the place on our bodies we naturally protect the most, and have been accustomed to doing so for a lifetime. Once you've done your first - and enjoyed the results - it really is a no-brainer.

Adam then told me to hold the swab on the site, as a compress, for a few seconds.

"Now, I'm going to leave you alone for five or ten minutes to self-stimulate, then I'll be back," Adam said. The door closed, and the lock turned so I wouldn't be interrupted.

There I sat, stimulating Mr. Floppy, coaxing him, stroking him, and nothing was happening. What am I doing sitting here on the ninth floor of a major New York City hospital, under garish lights, with nary a window, trying to masturbate? If my parents could see me now, came the thought. As they'd been dead for more than thirty years, I realized they probably were - and laughing heartily. This dulled my stimulating for a moment, then I told Mr. Floppy, "We can do this!"

By the time there was a knock on the door, my penis was hardly erect, but it was not - I repeat - not as lifeless as before. It was at once thrilling and disappointing. Then I remembered Adam speaking about starting off with the low dose.

Back in the room now, he examined me and asked how the results compared to my pre-surgery erections.

"About a third," I replied. Not in length, but in engorgement. As I continued to stand, though, things got a little happier down there. Not exciting, but yes, a little titillating. To feel the head of my penis now brushing against the cloth of my underwear was something I hadn't felt in six months. I giggled. Adam smiled and nodded his approval, adding, "A little gravity helps."

He also reminded me that if the effects lasted for more than four hours, to consult my doctor or local emergency room. Mr. Floppy returned about forty-five minutes later.

JAMIE: So what do you think, amigo?

MR. FLOPPY: I think this is great!

JAMIE: Didn't hurt, did it?

MR. FLOPPY: Hurt you way more than it did me. You looked, like, totally terrified, dude...

JAMIE: I was - but I did it.

MR. FLOPPY: Hello...? You may have rung the doorbell, but I opened the door.

JAMIE: So, you wouldn't mind doing this on a regular basis?

MR. FLOPPY: How soon does the kit get here?

JAMIE: I'll take that as a 'yes'. Adam said it would be about a week.

MR. FLOPPY: That's right. (PAUSE) Gonna be a long seven days...

JAMIE: Let's go home.

And we did. Injections continued, and the doses became larger until at 3.5 milliliters, we're pretty content.

The lesson here is don't be afraid of this therapy. It works. It doesn't give you the erection you had as a teenager, but how long ago was that anyway? It gives you not only the ability to penetrate and to pleasure your partner, but more importantly it gives you the feeling of being whole again - that there is life down there - and this is a very, very good feeling.

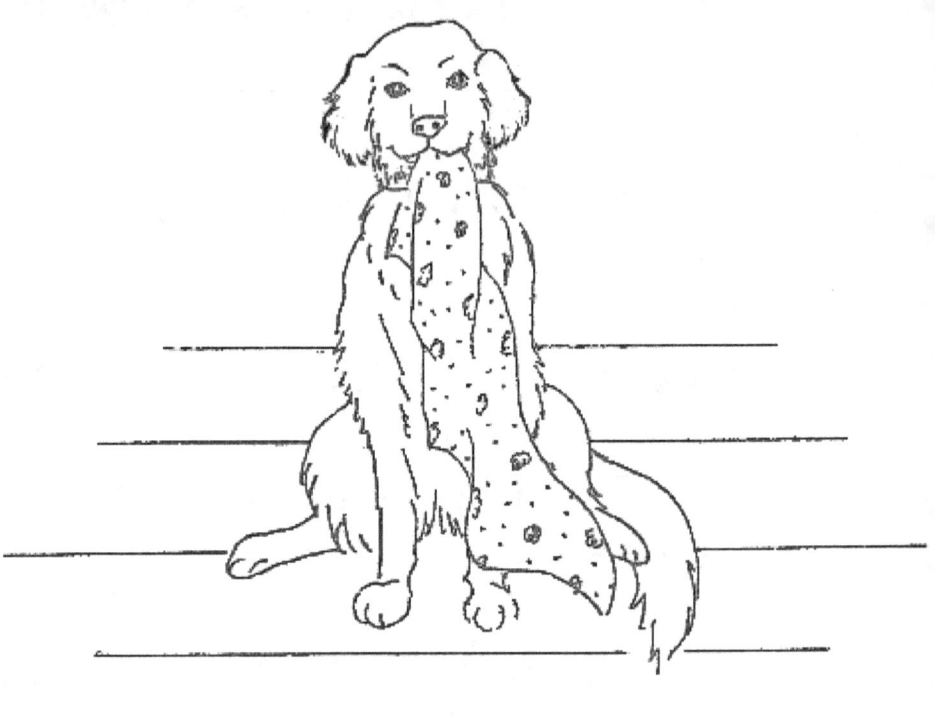

Chapter 14

RECALLED
TO LIFE

The first chapter of Charles Dickens' heartrending and haunting masterwork, *A Tale of Two Cities*, is titled "Recalled to Life." Doctor Manette, wrongly accused and long imprisoned in the Bastille, is rescued with the help of sympathetic friends determined to have him back in the bosom of his loving family in England.

"Buried how long?"
The answer was always the same.
"Almost eighteen years."
"You had abandoned all hope of being dug out?"

"Long ago."

"You know that you are recalled to life?"

"They tell me so."

The words were still in his hearing as just spoken - distinctly in his hearing as ever spoken words had been in his life - when the weary passenger started to the consciousness of daylight, and found that the shadows of the night were gone.

He lowered the window, and looked out at the rising sun. There was a ridge of ploughed land, with a plough upon it where it had been left last night when the horses were unyoked; beyond, a quiet coppice- wood, in which many leaves of burning red and golden yellow still remained upon the trees. Though the earth was cold and wet, the sky was clear, and the sun rose bright, placid, and beautiful.

MR. FLOPPY: Well, what was that all about?

JAMIE: Sorry, MF...?

MR. FLOPPY: I mean, how'd we get from 'stand-up happy soldier' and a sultry July day in Connecticut to November in the damp and cold English countryside - and don't say, "We flew."

JAMIE: Well, we're not literally in the...

MR. FLOPPY: And, also, you and your friend, Chuck, spelled the word 'plowed' wrong. And what the hell is a 'coppice-wood'?

JAMIE: Mr. Floppy...

MR. FLOPPY: Furthermore, at least when I last checked, we don't even have horses to unyoke, let alone -

JAMIE: MR. FLOPPY!!

MR. FLOPPY: What?

JAMIE: Will you please let me get a word in edgeways -

MR. FLOPPY: There you go again! It's 'edgewise'.

JAMIE: You're wrong. Both are correct. Now, hush.

MR. FLOPPY: (MUTTERING) Next thing you'll say is that I'm being a dickhead...

JAMIE: ENOUGH!! I added the excerpt from *A Tale of Two Cities* because it describes so eloquently, so poignantly, the feelings I've felt this past year -

MR. FLOPPY: ...WE'VE felt -

JAMIE: You interrupt me one more time, and the injection kit goes back!

MR. FLOPPY: (GULPING) ...yes, sir. (PAUSE) Uhmm, what do we do now...?

JAMIE: We ask them to turn the page.

MR. FLOPPY: How come?

JAMIE: Because we don't want them to miss the Postscript, coming up.

MR. FLOPPY: By the way, what are all the extra blank pages for at the end?

JAMIE: They're for making notes about doctors and services, for writing down questions, for listing important family and friends' phone contacts, and such.

My journey with prostate disease did not last eighteen long years - though, at times, it felt like a lifetime. I was not confined to a prison cell - though, at times, I felt wrongly accused and confined to cells of fear and dread. I was not in perpetual darkness - but did, at times, feel that normal, carefree light, as I knew it, would never quite be the same.

Some things, as you know them, will not be the same. This is good, and this is also somewhat sad. But this is life after prostate removal.

And although Mr. Floppy and I live argumentatively ever after, my sentimental reader...
...We Live.

POSTSCRIPT

Days before this book went to print, my 'twin', Dr. S. Ward 'Trip' Casscells III, born on the same day, in the same hospital as I was, lost his twelve-year war with prostate cancer.

He was an extraordinary person, led an extraordinary life, and touched an extraordinary number of people. Search his name online and you will readily see what a humble giant he was.

I knew him simply as Trippy and recall, early on, being somewhat confused as to why we lived in separate houses, since we looked so similar and celebrated our birthdays together every year.

A friend recently emailed a picture of him, taken at the summer camp in Maine we went to along with others from our home town of Greenville, Delaware. In the photograph there are three rows of us - black and white figures in shorts and T-shirts - staring at the camera, trying to look real cool (at age 12), me hoping the camera wouldn't notice my thick eyeglasses. Everyone looked at the lens, but Trippy. His gaze was somewhere else, not just at something that distracted him close by, but far away to a distant subject - something that puzzled and concerned him, his eyebrows slightly furrowed. Although he had a wonderful smile, the Trip I remember best was this Trip;

always intently fixed on solving a problem, or helping somebody - relentlessly giving himself to exploration, seeking answers and knowledge. Many called us old souls, compared to our contemporaries, which I think is true - especially being Pisces. But Trip was light years older than I, or anyone else I have ever known. This extreme, dual-edged gift gave him tremendous empathy for others. This sensitivity must also have caused him deep sorrow at times for all those he saw needing help. This made him a superb doctor and humanist.

When he was diagnosed with prostate disease, he threw himself into teamsmanship with the best minds available, and through five remissions gave of himself repeatedly, enthusiastically trying out conventional and unconventional therapies so that countless others, after him, might gain new knowledge and hope.

So, if he were typing this himself, I know he would write...

START TESTING AT 35 !

MORE ABOUT PROSTATE TRACKER

The ProstateTracker tools give each prostate cancer survivor an opportunity 'pay it forward' by helping other men find their prostate cancers early.

There are more than 240,000 new cases of prostate cancer diagnosed each year and 30,000 men die. But they don't need to die, they just need to know they have prostate cancer early, when it still is treatable.

One in six men will have prostate cancer. If each survivor gets six men to test and track using ProstateTracker, one of those men will have prostate cancer and a life just may be saved.

Please join the Prostate Cancer Awareness Project's "Just Get 6!" program.

WWW.PROSTATETRACKER.ORG

The description of Gleason scoring is reproduced with gracious permission of
John Wiley & Sons, Inc.

The description of the da Vinci prostatectomy is content of Intuitive Surgical, Inc
© 2012 Intuitive Surgical, Inc. Used with permission.

RAINDROPS KEEP FALLIN' ON MY HEAD
(from *Butch Cassidy & the Sundance Kid*)

RECALLED TO LIFE

_____

RECALLED TO LIFE

RECALLED TO LIFE

RECALLED TO LIFE

RECALLED TO LIFE

RECALLED TO LIFE

RECALLED TO LIFE

_____